Preparing for the Academic Foundation Programme: A Medical Student Handbook

Dr. Faisal Jamshaid
Dr. Miguel Sequeira Campos

In association with YoungAcademics and The Medical Education Foundation

ISBN: 9781709766817

CONTENTS

Preface

The Academic Foundation Programme (AFP) is the first stage at which doctors can benefit from dedicated research time alongside or in place of their clinical commitments. The purpose of this book is to provide a comprehensive overview of what the AFP is, why you should consider doing it, and how you can prepare for the various obstacles that stand in front of you as part of the application and interview processes.

The authors of this book were recently successful in their applications and were struck by the lack of readily available, high quality material for applicants to prepare for this competitive process. With this in mind, they have combined their knowledge of the programme with other successful applicants from across the UK to make a holistic, representative resource.

Passionate about medical education, the authors intended to create a high-yield resource for budding academics that would need no supplementation, and, have been striving to create high quality content that widens access for all backgrounds to develop a career in academic medicine.

N.B. The Authors have released this 1st edition copy primarily in an attempt to aid applicants of the 2020 AFP cycle approaching the interview stages. Therefore, this book has withheld advice and information on the preceding elements of the process, with all other sections to be included in the upcoming 2nd edition, in the run-up to the 2021 application cycle.

About the Authors

Dr. Faisal Jamshaid MBBS BSc (Hons)

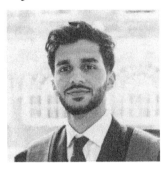

Faisal is currently an Academic Foundation Doctor (MedEd) at Basildon Hospital, Essex. He has published in high impact factor journals and presented his research internationally. During his time at King's College London, he founded Medtalk, Clinical Specialties Society and YoungAcademics, for which he was awarded a KCLSU Honorary Lifetime Membership. His interests include medical education, academic medicine and innovative solutions for healthcare professionals.

Dr. Miguel Sequeira Campos MBBS (Dist) BSc (Hons)

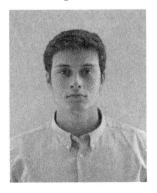

Miguel is currently an Academic Foundation Doctor in Plastic Surgery in London. He graduated from King's College with a First Class BSc in Anatomy and an MBBS degree with Triple Distinction and the medical school Gold Medal for highest ranking student. He has completed surgical fellowships at Harvard, Oxford and the National University of Singapore and is passionate about medical education and clinical research.

Contributors

Senior Reviewers

Mr Richmond James Colville
- Consultant Plastic Surgeon, St. George's Hospital, London

Mr Peter MacNeal MBChB BSc PgDip FHEA MRCS
- ST3 Plastic Surgeon, London

Dr Nga Nguyen MA (Cantab) MBBS AICSM
- Core Surgical Trainee Year 2, London

AFP Doctors

Dr Azeem Alam MBBS BSc (Hons)
- London AFP, Surgery at St Thomas' Hospital

Dr Shyam Gokani MBBS BSc
- London AFP, Primary Care and Population Health at University College London

Dr Xi Ming Zhu MBBS MSc BScH
- London AFP, General Practice at St. George's Hospital

Dr Eyal Ben-David, MBBS
- London AFP, Renal at St George's Hospital

Dr Saeed Azizi MBBS (Dist) Bsc (Hons)
- London AFP, General Practice at St George's Hospital

Dr Vageesh Jain MBBS MPH
- Leicester AFP, Public Health at NICE

Dr Rebecca Lissmann BA BMBS
- South West AFP, Leadership and Management

Dr Ciaran Kennedy MBChB MSc
- Yorkshire & Humber AFP, Medical Education at the University of Sheffield

Dr Harry Hodgson MBBS BSc
- Yorkshire & Humber AFP, Trauma & Orthopaedic Surgery

Dr Efioanwan Andah BSc MBBS
- Yorkshire and Humber AFP, Primary Care at Hull York Medical School

Dr Joseph P Thompson BSc (Hons) MB ChB
- West Yorkshire AFP, Neurosurgery at Leeds Teaching Hospitals Trust

Dr Saeed Azizi MBBS (Dist) Bsc (Hons)
- London AFP, General Practice at St George's Hospital

Chapter 1 - The Academic Foundation Programme

The Academic Foundation Programme (AFP) is an alternative route into training to the typical 'foundation programme' for doctors in the United Kingdom (UK). The main difference as compared with the regular foundation programme is the dedicated time to carry out research, develop leadership skills and even engage in teaching programmes. This typically occurs as a 4-month research block in Foundation Year 2 or in the form of 2-2.5 days every week (throughout the year) of protected time to carry out your academic duties.

This means that over the two foundation years, a typical junior doctor will have six clinical blocks (four months each). In comparison, an AFP doctor will have the five clinical placements and one academic block.

Each AFP 'post' will have a specific academic focus (e.g. cardiology, general surgery, medical education, etc.). In this way, an AFP doctor is afforded dedicated time in their field of interest to develop their research skills, work on a project and/or engage in teaching, leadership and other opportunities.

Contrary to popular belief, the AFP is not just for those who have a strong portfolio of publications and research presentations. It aims to introduce junior doctors to the idea of academic training pathways and, therefore, students can attain an AFP post without any prior academic experience - as long as they show a well-informed interest and some potential in academia. Nonetheless, AFP posts are very competitive and account for approximately 5% of foundation training posts in the country,

AFPs differ quite significantly in the way they are organised and by what they offer. It's important to familiarise yourself with the broad spectrum of posts to dispel preconceived notions of what an AFPs is limited to. It will also be important to have a firm understanding of the focus of the AFP you are applying for if you attend an interview.

As the academic component of the AFP is arranged with an associated university, you'll often be provided access to libraries, research support and other facilities. Additionally, with links to the university faculty, getting involved in teaching and other schemes becomes much more accessible.

Why choose the AFP?

There are numerous reasons why one may choose the AFP over the normal foundation programme. The first is fairly obvious: an interest in academic medicine. Another possible reason is to learn generic skills that aren't taught extensively in medical school (i.e. critical appraisal, manuscript drafting, presenting and critical thinking). Finally, applying for an AFP allows for additional foresight into potential placements and more independence in the shape of 'academic days'.

Alternatively, there are plenty of reasons why some decide that the AFP is not for them. As many applicants leave their decision to pursue the AFP to the last minute, it's often difficult to think clearly about the pros/cons amongst the busy hustle of final year. To make things easier, we've compiled a list of pros and cons of the AFP:

Positives

Dedicated research time - A four month block in year 2 dedicated to academic work. Alternatively, you may have an integrated block throughout the year. In this way, you have two sixth-month clinical placements with approximately two days off each week throughout the year for 'academic days'. There may be other commitments in these academic blocks specific to the AUoA (Academic Unit of Application)/Trust (e.g. on-call shift every other weekend, medical student teaching etc.) so look into this. As academic work is mostly independent, this also doubles up as a healthy break from clinical commitments.

Academic/general skill development - Work on academic skills such as literature searching, statistical analyses and manuscript drafting. In parallel, resulting academic presentations can further speaking, networking and presentation skills, an important skill-set for any career.

Know where you're going - Every AFP post will describe a pre-set combination of rotations and the hospital at which it will take place. These can be applied for as soon as foundation year applications open, alongside the normal FPAS route. While FPAS applicants have to be allocated a deanery before seeing a list of programmes/available rotations, AFP applicants can see exactly what they're applying for from the offset. This helps with getting to grips with application outcomes; you either get a post you specifically apply for, or no post at all.

Additional opportunities - AFP doctors often get the chance to undertake fully/partially funded post-graduate certifications (PGCERT), have easier access for ethical approval and even teaching opportunities. There may also provide easier access to university resources, library services, workspace and bursaries.

Negatives

Less clinical time - Achieving all the necessary competencies in F2 is often time-limiting, doing so in two-thirds of the time can be a tight squeeze! Additionally, one less clinical block means that you lose the opportunity to gain experience in as many fields as your peers.

Fixed rotations - When applying for an academic post, there is little room to exchange your clinical placements as they are predetermined by the trust. Therefore, in accepting an AFP post, you may be missing out on clinical rotations that you desire and accepting some that you dislike.

Less pay - Academic placements offer less pay than clinical placements (less hours, no on-calls etc.). Therefore, you may receive a slightly lower salary than that of your non-academic peers. However, it is easy to supplement this (if you so wish) by carrying out internal locuming at your hospital in F1 and locuming at your hospital or other hospitals in F2.

Same hospital for two years - Most AFPs will constitute a two-year programme at the same hospital. This may be a turn-off for those who wish to experience more than one hospital (often the combination of a district general hospital and a tertiary centre).

Scope for projects - A lot of AFPs have extremely niche academic focusses, particularly if your academic supervisor is keen on a certain subspecialty. This being said, some academic supervisors are happy for you to take the lead on you own desired topic, sometimes even letting you choose a whole different specialty!

Chapter 2 - The AFP Application

Below is a brief overview of the AFP timeline. Additional key dates can be found updated on the UKFP document 'Application Process Key Dates' each year by a quick look on www.foundationprogramme.nhs.uk or by a simple Google search. It's important to familiarise yourself with the key dates, particularly being aware of when: AFP posts are announced, applications are open and when interview invitations are rolled out (this information can be given on short notice).

Mon 23rd September 2019	Registration period opens. All programmes available to view on Oriel
Mon 30th September – Fri 11th October 2019 at 12:00	Application period for FP and AFP applications
From Mon 14th October 2019	AFP local short-listing and interview
Wed 15th January – 12th February 2020	AFP national and cascade offers
Thurs 12th March 2020	Primary list applicants informed of allocations

When selecting posts within an AUoA, there are several common approaches:

1. **Location** based. Some applicants are extremely keen to work in a particular hospital or area (particularly London and Oxford). These applicants may select every post in an AUoA, meaning that they'd be happy with any academic topic as long as it helps them to achieve a two-year post in a given place.
2. **Topic** based. E.g. If they're interested in vascular surgery, they'll simply apply for vascular surgery AFP posts, no matter the location within the AUoA. Most applicants usually adopt this approach, after first choosing an AUoA that they'd like to be based in.
3. **Clinical-block** based. Every AFP post has a predetermined set of clinical blocks. If having full foresight of your clinical blocks and hospital placement is something you'd like, it's worth a shot at applying for these AFP. You may even be able to change the

academic topic to something you'd prefer if you have a cool supervisor.

It's worth knowing about how the 'cascade process' works (the weeks following the first round of offers where subsequent offers are handed out for unfilled positions). If an AFP applicant rejects an offer from an AUoA (due to loss of interest, not replying within 48 hours or having accepted an offer from the alternative AUoA), this post will be offered to someone on the waiting list (applicants who reached interview stage but did not achieve a subsequent offer first time around). The cascade process lasts for three weeks after the initial round of offers. i.e. If the initial round of offers is on a Wednesday, the next three rounds of offers will take place on subsequent Wednesdays, with no offers being handed out in between. After these three weeks, no more offers are given out.

Applicants who are unsuccessful in the first round of offers may receive a 'change of application status' on the application portal (and email notification). This usually means that they are on the waiting list for subsequent rounds of offers. It's important to remember the 48 hour deadline to accept an offer. Failure to do so within the given time frame will lead to a **rejection** of the offer. Many students are either on elective placements or even regular holidays during this time. Difficulty gaining internet access in remote areas can lead to students being unable to accept offers in good time, pulling them out of the AFP process. Notably, any rejection of an AFP post (whether intentional or unintentional) will lead to complete withdrawal from that AUoA scheme (but not affecting your normal FP application).

It's worth noting that applying for only a select few posts has a unique advantage: you're more likely to receive an offer for those posts than those who select numerous additional posts. I.e. Some applicants receive an offer for a post they didn't really think through and end up rejecting it, resulting in a withdrawal from the cascade process. If they didn't add these additional 'filler' posts, they may have received an offer for their more preferential posts, albeit having to wait a few weeks longer in the cascade process.

Chapter 3 – General & Clinical Interview Stations

3.1 - Personal Questions & Ethical Scenarios

Personal questions are common in any interview, as you will likely have experienced when applying to medical school. They often allow applicants to convey their character whilst discussing their background and what they aspire to accomplish in the future. In the context of AFP interviews, the way they are used varies greatly between AUoAs. They may form the bulk of one of your stations, be mentioned at the beginning of one of your stations to place you at ease before you tackle the academic/ clinical scenarios, or they may not be used at all!

Ethical questions are less common in AFP stations but they do come up so it's worth being prepared. They may arise as an ethical scenario for you to discuss or simply as part of a larger clinical vignette (Ex. whilst you are on your way to see 2 unwell patients, you are asked by the police to provide information about one of your patients who has been stabbed and the nurse informs you a relative of one of your patients is phoning from abroad to ask about their clinical condition). At the very least, you should be aware of ethical and professional standards when dealing with common topics, such as capacity and confidentiality. Once you are comfortable with this, you should be able to outline and justify the steps you would take when confronted with an ethical scenario.

It is essential that frameworks are used to provide structured, slick answers with little preparation. You may choose to go through the sample questions provided below and prepare and memorise you own answers but this will likely be time-consuming and may come across as somewhat robotic during an interview. A fail-proof technique is to memorise a set of frameworks you can apply to most question types and then, think of examples for each category you are likely to be asked about.

After reading through the frameworks below, I recommend that you think about specific examples for each of the categories listed. You can then read through the worked examples to develop your understanding of how to tackle these questions. Finally, have a go at the worked examples provided in **Chapter 5**. You should practice answering these in front of friends/family and ask for their feedback. It is often difficult to strike a balance between selling yourself well and simply spewing cringey clichés -

so practice until you and those around you are happy that your answers put across your personality, achievements and aspirations in an effective and personal manner!

Frameworks

1. Questions asking you to provide a specific example of your experience to date = "**STARR**"
   - **Situation** - provide a background to how the situation arose
   - **Task** - outline what you set out to achieve
   - **Action** - highlight your role and the **skills** you employed or developed
   - **Result** - describe the end result of **your** action
   - **Reflection** - reflect on your learning points and how you will apply these to future situations, including the AFP. Focus especially on transferable skills you have developed

2. Questions asking about your background or where you see yourself heading in the future = "**CAMP**"
   - **Clinical** - Practice type (GP vs Hospital), Setting (DGH vs Tertiary Center), Particular specialty, Particular patient population, Experience you have/ hope to develop, etc.
   - **Academic** - Commitments (Full-time academic [Eg. PhD] vs Academic clinical role), Particular field of research, Particular lab of interest, etc.
   - **Management/leadership/teaching** - Taking part in MedTech, Teaching, Policy-making, Curriculum development, Managerial position in NHS, etc.
   - **Personal** - Provide some insight about your personal aspirations, which is a nice way to wrap up your answer in a personal and unique way

3. Questions asking about a challenging ethical scenario = "**SPIES**"
   - **Seek information** - from all parties, try and gain a good understanding of what took place, is this an isolated episode or a pattern, are there 2 sides to the scenario
   - **Patient safety** - ensure that patients are kept safe as your highest priority
   - **Initiative** - carry out any suitable actions yourself before escalating
   - **Escalate** - seek advice from colleagues or seniors, as appropriate

- **Support** - ensure those involved feel supported, as well as patients and the team

General Question Categories

The following categories are likely to arise during AFP interviews. It would be prudent to prepare a few examples of your achievements in each category that you would like to bring up if asked.

1. Motivation for an AFP/ Academic career
2. Motivation for an AFP at THAT deanery
3. Good clinical practice
4. Research experience
5. Teaching experience
6. Teamwork experience
7. Leadership experience
8. Extracurriculars/ Volunteering experience
9. Strengths
10. Weaknesses
11. Obstacles overcome

The following are common categories for ethical scenario questions:

1. Capacity
2. Confidentiality
3. Punctuality
4. Poor team-work/ leadership
5. Patient safety concerns with a colleague/ senior

3.2 - The Clinical Emergencies Station

The clinical station is mainly designed to test your ability to manage an acutely unwell patient. Nevertheless, there are various other skills and knowledge that the examiners will be assessing, such as your ability to prioritise and escalate appropriately.

In the clinical station, you may be presented with a vignette for a single acutely unwell patient or various unwell patients. You will be expected to discuss your initial approach, including investigations and management. If you have more than one patient to discuss, you will be expected to prioritise and justify your decisions.

In this handbook, we will first go over the theoretical knowledge you will require. We will then talk through various examples. Finally, you will encounter several vignettes for you to practice with friends before your interview. For maximum benefit, we recommend that you practice these under timed conditions that replicate what you will encounter on your interview day. If your AUoA doesn't provide information about timings we recommend you practice for a 10-15 minute station.

Key Background Knowledge

"Continuous monitoring" refers to a set of observations, including:
- Respiratory rate
- Oxygen saturations
- Blood pressure
- Heart rate
- 3-lead ECG (also known as "cardiac monitor")

When dealing with acutely unwell patients, it is often a good idea to suggest that you would request the nurses responsible for the patient carry out "continuous monitoring" whilst you carry out your assessment of the patient.

"Early Warning Scores (EWS)" are dynamic, standardised scoring systems that attribute points to particular ranges of vital signs, allowing you to monitor patients' progression. Ex. The National Early Warning System (**NEWS**) is used preferentially in the UK

		Score						
ABCDE	**PARAMETER**	3	2	1	0	1	2	3
Airway & Breathing	**Respiratory Rate (breaths/min)**	≤8		9-11	12-20		21-24	≥25
	SpO2 (%)	≤91	92-93	94-95	≥96			
	In hypercapnic respiratory failure where target sats are 88-92%	≤83	84-85	86-87	≥93 (on air) 88-92 (on O2)	93-94 on O2	95-96 on O2	≥97 on O2
	Air vs Oxygen		Oxygen		Air			
Circulation	**Systolic BP (mmHg)**	≤90	91-100	101-110	111-129			≥220
	Heart rate (beats/min)	≤40		41-50	51-90			≥131
Disability	**Consciousness (AVPU)**				Alert			New onset confusion/ Voice/ Pain/ Unresponsive
Exposure	**Temperature (°C)**	≤35.0		35.1-36.0	36.1-38.0	38.1-39.0	≥39.1	

13

Response to NEWS Scores:

Score	Minimum monitoring frequency	Action
0	12 hourly	Continue routine monitoring
1-4 in total	4-6 hourly	Registered nurse to assess patient & decide monitoring/ escalation
3 in single parameter	1 hourly	Registered nurse to inform medical team + medical team to review & decide
5-6 tota (Urgent response)	1 hourly	Registered nurse to immediately inform medical team + medical team to urgently review & decide
7+ total (Emergency response)	Continuous	Registered nurse to immediately inform medical team + medical minimum SpR to review & consider transfer to level $2/3$ care (HDU, ICU)

Handover — you could be asked to provide a handover to a colleague over the phone. Handovers are used extremely frequently in hospital when referring to different specialties, reporting back to your seniors or passing over responsibility for patient care at the end of your shift. Having a structure to provide a handover is very important and the **SBAR** approach is most commonly used.

> **Situation** - identify (1) who you are (2) the patient you're calling about and why
> **Background** - outline (1) the patient's admission (2) relevant Past Medical Hx
> **Assessment** - provide (1) NEWS score or vital signs (2) your clinical assessment - which is often structured in an ABCDE format for acute patients (see below)
> **Recommendation** - cover (1) what you think should happen to the patient (2) what you need from them (3) whether there is anything you can do to help them (4) confirm what they will do and when (5) Thank them

Ex. Here is a scenario of a doctor feeling overwhelmed and requesting help from a senior. Notice that despite an incomplete

ABCDE assessment, he manages to come across as professional through a structured handover.

> Situation - (1) My name is John and I'm the F1 on-call in Gray Ward calling for the Medical Registrar. (2) I am calling about Mr Smith, a 75 year old male in Bed 22, Hospital number 12345. 20 minutes ago he became acutely short of breath with his saturations dropping to 90% on room air, a RR of 24 and a HR of 110.
>
> Background - (1) He underwent an elective hip replacement yesterday. (2) He has a background of high blood pressure and well controlled asthma.
>
> Assessment - (1) I have started the patient on 15L of oxygen via a non-rebreather mask, sent off various bloods and requested a portable CXR. I'm about to carry out an ECG. The patient's vitals are: SpO2 has since gone up to 93% on 15L of O2, RR is now 19, HR is now 100, BP 120/90, Temp 37.2 and he is currently alert. (2) I completed a partial A-E assessment but I'm worried he is deteriorating rapidly.
>
> Recommendation - (1) I think this patient has either developed a PE or respiratory sepsis but am unable to rule out other causes, such as cardiac. (2) I would really appreciate it if you could help me review him as I feel out of my depth. (3) Is there anything you recommend I do in the meantime? (4) So can I confirm you will be here within 15 minutes? (5) Thank you.

Escalation/ Support - It is very important to know who you can turn to for help in different situations. You will require this knowledge as a doctor and, as such, you will be tested on your awareness of escalation pathways during your AFP interview. Here are some rules of thumb:

- **General**
  - **Cardiac arrest** - put out a cardiac arrest call ("crash call") on 2222 and shout for someone to bring the "crash" or cardiac arrest trolley as you start CPR (it is unlikely this will be one of your scenarios but it is still useful to be aware of)
  - **Critically unwell patient about to arrest** - put out a peri-arrest call on 2222 (or call for the Medical Emergency Team [also referred to as a "MET Call"])
  - **Critically unwell patient not about to arrest** - critical care outreach team (this is often a team of highly

specialised nurses who provide ITU expertise/ patient assessment for ITU to other wards in the hospital)

- **Airway**
  - ○ **Concerns about patient maintaining airway** - either put out a cardiac arrest call (includes an anaesthetist) or call your hospital switchboard through 2222 and ask them to fast-bleep the anaesthetist
- **Breathing**
  - ○ **Medical issues** - you can seek help from the Medical Registrar or "MedReg"
  - ○ **Ventilation** - if you require Non-invasive ventilation (Ex. with a COPD patient in Type 2 Respiratory failure before intubation) you can call the critical care outreach team
- **Circulation**
  - ○ **Medical conditions out of hours** - bleep the Medical Registrar
  - ○ During the working day, here is a list of specialties to contact for common conditions:
    - ▪ **Cardiology** - ACS, Acute HF, Severe HTN, Infective Endocarditis, Arrhythmia
    - ▪ **Dermatologists** - worrying rash, skin emergency (Eg. TEN, SJS)
    - ▪ **Endocrinology** - DKA, HHS, Addisonian crisis, Cushing's, Pheochromocytoma, Thyroid disease
    - ▪ **Gastroenterology** - Upper GI bleed, Severe diarrhoea
    - ▪ **Gynaecologists** - vaginal bleeding, suspected ovarian/ uterine/ vaginal pathology
    - ▪ **Haematology** - Disseminated Intravascular Coagulation/
    - ▪ **Microbiology** - sepsis
    - ▪ **Nephrology** - Severe AKI, Nephrotic/ nephritic syndromes, Poor urine output
    - ▪ **Neurology** - stroke, meningitis, coma, UMN/ LMN signs/ symptoms
    - ▪ **Obstetricians** - acutely unwell pregnant woman
    - ▪ **Orthopaedics** - trauma, septic arthritis
    - ▪ **Respiratory** - TB, severe pneumonia
    - ▪ **Rheumatology** - acute mono/ polyarthritis
    - ▪ **Surgeons** - haemorrhage, acute abdomen

Remember your basic algorithms (BLS, ALS) - it is unlikely you will be required to bring this up in the context of an interview but it is good to be aware of so you understand how a situation may change when seeing an unwell patient. The general rules to remember are:

- Unwell patient = ABCDE Assessment
- Unresponsive patient? = BLS/ ALS depending on your level of training (NOTE: most of you have NOT done ALS training so this will NOT be expected - you can skip this section)

If you are conducting an ABCDE assessment on a patient and they stop responding, you must start your BLS/ ALS algorithm. Remember "DRS ABCC"

BLS (Unconscious patient)

1. **Danger** - assess whether it is safe to manage this patient (Ex. fire, electric cables, etc.).
2. **Response** - assess the patient's response to pain by calling for them clearly in each ear. If they do not respond, assess their response to pain with a trapezius squeeze.
3. **Shout** for help
4. Airway -
5. Breathing - for 10 seconds you must Look (chest movement), Listen (breaths), Feel (breaths) - you can feel for a carotid pulse at the same time
6. Call - 999 (out-of-hospital) 2222 (in-hospital) - State: where you are; what you need (adult cardiac arrest call; obstetric cardiac arrest call)
7. Chest compressions - start chest compressions at a rate of 30 compressions: 2 rescue breaths (this is the algorithm for adult life support, it is different for children/ neonates)

ALS (If you are appropriately trained and have access to a defibrillator)
1. Attach defibrillator pads (WITHOUT interrupting chest compressions)
2. Assess rhythm & pulse
    a. Shockable (Ventricular Fibrillation/ pulseless Ventricular Tachycardia)
        i. 1mg IV Adrenaline + 300mg IV Amiodarone - after 3rd and 5th shock
        ii. 1mg IV Adrenaline - every alternate cycle thereafter
    b. Non-shockable (Asystole/ Pulseless Electrical Activity with NO pulse)
        . 1mg IV Adrenaline - as soon as you obtain IV access
        i. 1mg IV Adrenaline - every alternate cycle thereafter
3. Start ruling out the causes of reversible cardiac arrest (4Hs and 4Ts)
    - Hypovolemia - give IV fluid bolus
    - Hypoxia - give 15L 100% O2 via NRB mask
    - Hypo/hyperkalaemia - Check U&Es, ABG
    - Hypothermia - Check temperature
    - Tamponade - Auscultate the heart, check the JVP/ BP, order focused cardiac USS
    - Tension pneumothorax - auscultate/ percuss for bilateral air entry, check that the trachea is central
    - Thromboembolism - check legs, auscultate
    - Toxins - review drug chart

3.3 - The ABCDE Assessment

The goal of the ABCDE assessment is to stabilise the acutely unwell patient. This is accomplished by working through the most important systems and correcting abnormalities as you encounter them (Ex. administering oxygen for low O2 sats and high RR or administering IV fluids for low BP, etc.) Once you commit the ABCDE approach to memory, you should never miss anything crucial when managing an unwell patient (or talking about how to manage one in an interview).

My advice would be to read through the components of the ABCDE assessment included below (alongside pathologies certain findings can suggest) and try to commit them to memory. You can then start thinking about applying these to different clinical scenarios. Eventually, once you are comfortable, you can remember the fine details for individual clinical conditions which we have included below.

Remember: the aim of this station is to ensure you are a safe FY1 - don't get sidetracked trying to showcase your theoretical medical knowledge (Eg. with specific 4th line drug doses and doses of thrombolytic agents to administer) whilst forgetting the very basic things. [I.e. Don't obsess about memorising doses of vasopressors for acute refractory heart failure - it is highly unlikely you would ever be doing this in clinical practice! Likewise, even if you are pretty confident your patient has respiratory sepsis, you must still carry out a BM reading - never forget the simple things which are those that an F1 is expected to know!]

Before we go into further detail regarding the ABCDE assessment, remember what you would be expected to do when faced with an unwell patient as a junior doctor:

1. Before you see your patient: obtain an appropriate SBAR handover (see above)
2. If possible ask a nursing colleague to grab the patient notes and meet you by the bedside so they can assist you
3. Introduce yourself to the patient and carry out a full ABCDE assessment, correcting abnormalities as you encounter them. Every time you correct an abnormality, you should restart your ABCDE assessment (don't do this in an interview as you waste valuable time but make sure you convey that you are aware of this)
4. After you are happy the patient is stable, approach them as you would with a stable patient
   a. Take a full clinical history

b. Carry out necessary examinations

c. Consider further laboratory or radiological investigations

d. Review the patient notes fully and come up with a management plan

5. Document your encounter with the patient

6. Discuss you plan with a senior and handover to any relevant parties (Ex. the night team, a senior colleague or even a different team who need to see the patient)

Now let's look at each of the components of the ABCDE Assessment in a little more detail...

AIRWAY (Remember "AC" for "Airway, C-spine")

- When you arrive at the bedside: Introduce yourself to the patient and ask "How are you?" If the patient replies to you, you can assume their airway is patent. Otherwise, assess their airway and consider simple interventions to secure the airway until the anaesthetist arrives to protect it with an Endotracheal (ET) tube.
- Inspect inside the mouth for visible obstructions, which you can remove by suction (Yankauer sucker) or with Magill forceps (curved forceps - only use under direct vision if comfortable!)
  - Airway manoeuvres
    - Head tilt and chin lift
    - Jaw thrust
  - Airway adjuncts
    - Nasopharyngeal airway
    - Oropharyngeal airway (Guedel) - Note: if your patient tolerates an OP airway, this is an indication that their GCS is likely ≤8 (indication for intubation) - you **must** call an anaesthetist (2222 crash call OR 2222 to get switchboard to fastbleep anaesthetist)
    - iGel (Supraglottic airway)
    - Laryngeal mask airway
    - Endo-tracheal tube (Inserted by an anaesthetist; protects against aspiration)
  - If you believe the patient may have sustained a cervical-spinal injury you should:
    1. Suggest C-spine protection through 3-point spinal immobilisation (collar, bags, tape) as per ATLS guidelines
    2. Jaw-thrust (not head-tilt, chin-lift) to maintain the airway

NB: *this is unlikely to come up in your interview but it is good to be aware*

BREATHING

- **RR** - count the patient's respiratory rate, a valuable indication of whether a patient is unwell
  - Low RR - opioids, sedation, raised ICP, life-threatening asthma
  - High RR - asthma, COPD, sepsis, pneumonia, pneumothorax, pulmonary oedema, heart failure, anxiety, PE

- **IPPA** - Carry out a simple chest exam by Inspection, Palpation, Percussion, Auscultation
  - **Inspect** - for signs of respiratory distress (central cyanosis, accessory muscle use, see-saw breathing with abdominal movement in laboured breaths)
  - **Palpate** - bilateral chest expansion (unequal in fibrosis, tension pneumothorax, consolidation); subcutaneous emphysema (feels like Rice Krispies under the skin)
  - **Percuss** - equal bilateral chest expansion; tracheal deviation (tension pneumothorax); hyper-resonance may suggest a pneumothorax, dullness may suggest consolidation/ pleural effusion/ atelectasis
  - **Auscultate** - bronchial breathing in consolidation; reduced breath sounds in pneumothorax/ pleural fluid/ complete obstruction of airways by lung consolidation
- **Arterial Blood Gas**
  - Suggest an ABG if the patient is showing signs of respiratory distress
  - Not that someone will have to take this to the nearest ABG machine for results
  - Will give you blood pH, PO2, PCO2, HCO3, Base excess, O2 sats, Na+, K+, Ca2+, Cl-, Lactate
  - It is also useful to look at COHb (a patient with headache/ reduced consciousness could have Carbon Monoxide poisoning)
- **Oxygen saturations**
  - Consider attaching an oxygen saturation probe
  - Most patients have target saturations 94-98% - if below this, you can start them on Oxygen
  - Most unwell patients are started on 15L of 100% Oxygen via a Non-rebreather mask (NRB)

- o If a patient is a known CO_2 retainer and target saturations are 88-92%
  - If they are unwell hypoxia will kill them before hypercapnia therefore start them on 15L of Oxygen via NRB and do an ABG to see if they are in Type 2 Respiratory Failure (i.e. Retaining CO_2) - if so, you can then switch them to a fixed performance Venturi mask
  - o If a patient is requiring more than 15L NRB or is in Type 2 Respiratory failure (Low PO2, high CO_2) they may require Non-invasive Ventilation (call ITU outreach) or intubation (fast-bleep an anaesthetist or put out a crash call)
- **Chest X-Ray**
  - o Necessary if you suspect lung pathology. Could be arranged as a portable scan with the Radiographers if the patient is too unwell to travel to the X-ray department
- **Needle decompression**
  - o To be carried out immediately if you suspect a tension pneumothorax (Tracheal deviation, Hyper-resonance or reduced breath sounds on 1 side - this is a clinical Dx, don't wait for imaging confirmation)
  - o 2nd Intercostal space Midclavicular line (alternatively, 5th ICS Midaxillary Line)
- **Nebulisers**
  - o If the patient is wheezing you can consider nebulisers to provide relief - the type of nebulisers will depend on the pathology you suspect or level of senior support you have (Ex. salbutamol for asthma, nebulised adrenaline as an adjunct to the emergency treatment for anaphylaxis - see below)

CIRCULATION
- **A good way to remember the main points to consider in Circulation is to start at the fingertips and travel up the arm (Temp, CRT, Radial Pulse, BP, JVP, Mucous membranes, Heart, ECG). You can then consider further interventions: IV access ± bloods ± intravenous fluid administration; catheterisation to monitor urine output (surrogate for kidney function); cross-match or group & save (if the patient is likely to require a blood transfusion); ECG (often done for unwell patients)**
- Temperature

- o   Are the patient's limbs warm and well perfused or cold and peripherally shut down?
  - o   You can also inspect the colour of the hands
- **Capillary Refill Time**
  - o   Press the patient's nailbeds for 5 seconds and release - a normal peripheral circulation would see the colour return in <2 seconds
  - o   Long CRT can suggest the patient is peripherally shut down: shock or dehydration
- **Radial Pulse**
  - o   Rate? Rhythm? (Irregularly irregular in Atrial Fibrillation) Character?
  - o   Does the pulse feel bounding (sepsis, Aortic Regurgitation), nice and strong (normal) or weak and thready (poor cardiac output)?
  - o   Radial-radial delay in aortic coarctation/ dissection
- **Blood Pressure**
  - o   High BP in PE, fluid overload, endocrine causes, etc.
  - o   Low BP in haemorrhage, hypovolemia, sepsis, etc.
- **Jugular Venous Pressure**
  - o   Can be high in severe asthma, heart failure, fluid overload, cardiac tamponade
- **Mucous membranes**
  - o   Does the patient look dehydrated?
- **Heart**
  - o   Auscultate for heart murmurs and remember:
    - ▪   Murmur + unknown pyrexia = you MUST exclude infective endocarditis
    - ▪   Pericardial rub in pericarditis
    - ▪   S3 - volume overload
    - ▪   S4 - pressure overload
- **ECG**
  - o   Carry out a 12-lead ECG. Compare it with a previous ECG if one exists. If you are unsure what it shows, you could ask the Medical Registrar/ Cardiologist for advice
- **IV access**
  - o   If a patient is very unwell it may be prudent to insert 2 large bore cannulae (14-16G)
    - ▪   A good way to remember colours and sizes imagining travelling outwards from the centre of the Earth (read below, before you judge...):
      - •   Earth's core is Orange = 14G
      - •   Rocky surface of the Earth is Grey = 16G

- - - The grasslands at the surface are Green = 18G
    - The flowers over the grass are Pink = 20G
    - The sky is Blue = 22G
    - The sun is Yellow = 24G
    - The galaxies can be seen as Purple = 26G
- **Blood results**
  - Full Blood Count
    - Hb - anaemia
    - White Cell Count - infection
  - Urea & Electrolytes + Creatinine
  - Liver function Tests + Amylase
  - Troponin
  - D-dimer
  - C-reactive protein
  - Brain Natriuretic Peptide (BNP)
  - Endocrine tests
  - Drug screen
  - Blood cultures - essential in sepsis
- **Intravenous fluids**
  - If the patient is septic or appears dehydrated with low BP, you can administer a fluid bolus and monitor the response. Use a crystalloids: either Sodium chloride 0.9% (normal saline) or Hartmann's
    - 500ml of 0.9% Sodium Chloride administered over 15 minutes
    - 250ml of 0.9% Sodium Chloride administered over 15 minutes - in patients with heart failure, elderly/ frail
- **Catheterisation**
  - A catheter will allow you to monitor the patient's urine output
  - URINALYSIS
    - **And pregnancy test in ALL FEMALES**
- **Cross-match/ Group & Save**
  - If you believe the patient will likely need a blood transfusion or will be going to theatre for a procedure where there is significant anticipated blood loss

DISABILITY
- **Glucose**
- **Pupils**

- o (1) Appearance: Size, Symmetry (2) Reaction to Light/ Accommodation
- o A lack of reaction to light/ accommodation may indicate pathology in the visual system or brain (stroke, cerebral compression from blood/ trauma)
    - Pupil reflexes intact = midbrain intact
    - Small pupils in opioid overdose (administer antagonist Naloxone) or pontine pathology
    - Unilaterally dilated and unreactive pupil = Cranial nerve III lesion (DM or Posterior Communicating Artery aneurysm)
    - Horner's = consider ipsilateral medullary/ hypothalamic lesion
- **Glasgow Coma Score (A simpler alternative is the AVPU score)**
    - o **Remember EVM, 456 - the minimum score is 3** (deep coma, death)
        - Eye opening
            - 1 = none
            - 2 = opens eyes to pain
            - 3 = opens eyes to voice
            - 4 = spontaneous eye opening
        - Verbal response
            - 1 = none
            - 2 = inappropriate sounds
            - 3 = inappropriate words
            - 4 = confused
            - 5 = normal, oriented
        - Motor response
            - 1 = none
            - 2 = Extension to pain (Decerebrate, Lesion involving Red nucleus)
            - 3 = Flexion to pain (Decorticate, Lesion above Red nucleus)
            - 4 = Withdraws from pain (will move away from trapezius squeeze)
            - 5 = Localises to pain (will remove your hand in a trapezius squeeze)
            - 6 = normal, follows commands
    - o A GCS ⩽8 warrants airway protection by an ET-tube
    - o NOTE: Midbrain's **<u>red nucleus</u>** reinforces flexion and loss of red nucleus = limb extension

- **Central Nervous System**
    - ○ Consider simplified Cranial Nerve/ Upper limb/ Lower limb neurological examinations if you suspect a neurological pathology

EXPOSURE
- **Expose**
    - ○ Ensure curtains are drawn to preserve dignity. Fully expose the patient & inspect the body - including the back as well as bottom and genital region
- **Temperature**
    - ○ Record the patient's temperature
- **Analgesia**
    - ○ Ensure the patient has adequate analgesia
- **Antibiotics**
    - ○ If you believe the patient is septic, remember your "Sepsis Six" - including broad spectrum antibiotics until you have culture results and discuss with microbiology to narrow the spectrum
    - ○ If you don't know which antibiotics are usually administered for a particular condition it is often safe to say you would check the Micro Guide for your local policy. This is actually the best way to do things in clinical practice too as local sensitivities vary depending on the patient population!

As you work through each of the examples below, you can add/ remove different components as you see fit. The goal is to stabilise the patient and arrive at a sensible differential diagnosis in order to start implementing further management.

Now let's apply this framework to the context of an interview...

If you are given a scenario with a single patient, follow the steps outlined above and remember to include
1. your list of differential diagnoses
2. How you would narrow down this list by investigating appropriately
3. How you would manage the patient/ Who you would refer to

If you are given a scenario with multiple unwell patients, you should start by acknowledging this:

1. In this scenario, there are 2 unwell patients
2. My priority is patient safety and I would escalate to my seniors (even if they are unable to help right now) to make them aware of the situation
3. I would then see patient 1 because… (provide a justification as to why you believe this patient is more acutely unwell)
4. However, in the meantime, I would ask my colleagues to do the following…

   Remember, even if you are seeing patient 1, the nurse who will likely have called you to see patient 2 will be able to do many things to help you once you see the second patient. If patient 2 is unwell, you could consider suggesting

   - A full set of observations, to be repeated every 15 minutes until you see the patient
   - Continuous monitoring (see above)
   - Giving the patient oxygen (this should technically be prescribed beforehand but no-one will deprive a breathless patient of oxygen if you are unable to prescribe it immediately)
   - Remind your colleagues that if the patient deteriorates and they become increasingly worried, they can put our a peri-arrest call!

Some tips for the interview:
BEFORE THE STATION

If you are given time before the interview to read through the vignette, use it wisely! This is how we would recommend you use any time you have:

1. Read through the vignette and underline the key information from each clinical scenario - Eg. patient gender, age, past medical history, observations, etc.
2. Write a brief ABCDE assessment along the margin and fill this out with any information you will want to gather and what interventions you may consider. This will ensure that in the fast-paced environment of the interview room, you won't forget to mention anything important.
3. If there is more than 1 consideration (Ex. multiple unwell patients), write down who you will see first and why.

DURING THE STATION

My first tip would be to remember to slow down and think before you say anything. It is perfectly fine to take your time and pause and this will make you come across as a calm and composed medical student who is ready to face stressful emergency situations as a doctor.

Remember to always ask for help early and put patient safety first! There may be more you can do for your patient before calling for senior help but, if you get the impression they are deteriorating fast, it is best to inform someone more experienced. You can always inform a senior of the patient's current condition and then make them aware of the steps you will be taking until they come and review.

Remember you are never alone in the hospital. There are nurses, colleagues at the same level, senior members of your team and other seniors you can call. You cannot exist in two places at once, which means if there are 2 patients who require immediate medical attention, someone else will have to see one of them - whether this is an F1 colleague, Senior House Office "SHO" (FY2, CT1/2), Registrar (ST3+) or even Consultant. If one of the patients is less unwell, you can ask a nursing colleague to carry out jobs they are qualified to do to save you time whilst you see your first patient (nurses can measure vital signs or start a breathless patient on oxygen and they can often take bloods, insert catheters and cannulae, etc. These are all jobs you will likely require when assessing an unwell patient and so your nursing colleagues can be of great assistance when things get very busy.).

AFTER THE STATION

After you are done with the station, try not to worry about your performance. This is especially important if you have an academic station immediately after. The worst that could happen would be to replay the station in your head and lose focus for the next station.

If you leave feeling like it went terribly: I feel compelled to remind you that, as in many aspects of our lives, we are our own harshest critics. Myself and other applicants who scored maximum points in the clinical station left thinking it had gone terribly. All you will likely remember are the points that you did not mention and the conditions you did not consider.

If you leave feeling like it went great: That's great news! But don't get complacent. Take time to reflect if you can and then move on. Focus on your next station, your next interview or your next set of exams. If this was your last hurdle this year, enjoy your well deserved rest.

Let's look at some specific clinical scenarios…

N.B. For this first edition, we have aimed to make this section as concise as possible. This means we have omitted some basic information in favour of more advanced information. Do not panic if you find some of the management too advanced. You are NOT expected to memorise everything we have included here and your focus should be on doing the basic ABCDE assessment well - showing you have enough knowledge to be a safe and competent AFP doctor.

Your approach should be to:
1. Go through an ABCDE assessment, including the standard management you would apply to any situation (Eg. Oxygen for low saturation, Fluids in low BP + dehydration, ECG in suspected chest pathology)
2. Use the management listed below to show more advanced knowledge

Remember that simply going through the standard ABCDE management would suffice to stabilise most patients until senior support arrives. Anything you show beyond that is good as it will show you are functioning above the level which is expected of you. Having said that, remember your limitations - Eg. even if you know pacing is the most appropriate next step in the bradycardia algorithm, that does not mean you will carry it out without appropriate ALS training. Acknowledge this! **Say: "After Atropine administration the patient remains bradycardic so I would immediately summon a senior with a view to implementing more advanced management, which could include further atropine doses/ transcutaneous pacing/ or other drugs such as IV isoprenaline or adrenaline. This would be a senior led decision and I would provide support within the limits of my clinical competency"**

Some common presentations to consider:

1. **Headache and...**
   - **Thunderclap? First and worst?** - think Subarachnoid haemorrhage (consider referring to Neurology)
   - **Unilateral** - think Migraine, Cluster headache, Acute angle closure glaucoma (refer to Ophthalmology for urgent tonometry for intraocular pressure), rule out Giant Cell arteritis (refer to Ophthalmology)
   - **Worse when straining/ coughing/ bending/ early in the morning** - think raised ICP/ venous thrombosis (order a CT, consider referring to Neurosurgery)

- **Scalp tenderness** - think Giant Cell arteritis (Get an ESR + refer to Ophthalmology urgently for initiation of steroid administration)
- **Fever/ Photophobia/ Phonophobia/ Neck stiffness** - think meningitis (In the community give IM BenPen, in hospital start IV Ceftriaxone ± Ampicillin)
- **Pregnancy** - think pre-eclampsia (Check BP, Urine dip for protein, Refer to Obstetrics)
- **Foreign travel** - think malaria (get your blood films)
- **Reduced consciousness** - think stroke, space occupying lesion (tumour/ abscess), haemorrhage (subdural, extradural, subarachnoid), venous thrombosis, meningitis

2.   **Shortness of Breath and...**
- **Vesicular breath sounds** - think Cardiac cause (Ex. ACS), Pulmonary Embolism, Anxiety (hyperventilation), Diabetic Ketoacidosis, Shock, Salicylate overdose, Pneumocystis jirovecii (PCP) pneumonia commonly in HIV patients
- **Stridor** - foreign body or traumatic obstruction (Ex. laryngeal fracture), epiglottitis, croup, laryngomalacia (often in children), bacterial tracheitis, anaphylaxis
- **Wheezing** - think AABBCC → Asthma, Bronchiolitis, Bronchiectasis, COPD, Cardiac (HF)
- **Crepitations/ Crackles** - pneumonia, fibrosis, heart failure, bronchiectasis (thick secretions)
- **Stony dull percussion** - pleural effusion
- **Chest Pain** - think cardiac cause, pneumonia, pneumothorax (hyperresonance)
- **Arrhythmia on ECG** - may require immediate cardioversion, liaise with seniors/ cardiology

3.   **Chest pain**
- **Cardiac** (often dull/ crushing/ associated with exertion) - Stable angina (relieved by rest), Unstable angina (not relieved by rest), NSTEMI (troponin elevation at 6h or 12h), STEMI (ST elevation 1mm limb leads, 2mm chest leads), Pericarditis
- **Respiratory** (often sharp) - Pulmonary Embolism (CTPA), Pneumothorax (CXR) Pneumonia (CXR)
- **Aortic dissection** (CT/MRI)
- **Oesophageal** - GORD, Oesophagitis (endoscopic finding), Oesophageal rupture

- **Musculoskeletal** (tenderness on **palpation** of chest wall) - Muscular, Rib #, Costochondritis (or Tietze's if costal cartilage swelling)
- **Psychiatric** - panic attack

4. **Upper abdominal pain**
   - GORD - endoscopy
   - Biliary colic, Cholecystitis (pain + fever), Cholangitis (Charcot's triad: pain + fever + jaundice)
   - Pancreatitis
   - Remember - a cardiac/ respiratory cause can present as upper abdominal pain!

5. **Reduced consciousness**
   - **Neurological**
     - **Trauma**
     - **Infection** - meningitis, encephalitis, malaria
     - **Vascular -** stroke, bleed (subdural, extradural, subarachnoid)
     - **Space occupying lesion** - tumour, abscess
   - **Metabolic**
     - **Septic-like but no fever** - think Addisonian crisis
     - **Overdose**

3.4 – ABCDE -Worked Examples

Unconscious patient
    A. 15L O2/ Stabilise c-spine if cause could be trauma

    B. RR for overdose (Opiates, Benzos) / Respiratory pattern (Cheyne-Stokes = brainstem lesion/ compression from oedema; Hyperventilation in DKA; Apneustic breathing in brainstem damage) / ABG for Lactate (Sepsis) + COHb + Electrolytes

    C. BP hypertensive encephalopathy / Bloods for Alcohol, Salicylate, Paracetamol, LFTs, U&Es, TFTs, Cortisol, Glucose, Pregnancy, Troponin, D-dimer

    D. Pupils for stroke, opiates / Glucose for hypo / GCS to quantify severity + airway protection / Neuro exam for localising lesions (test tone, reflexes)

    E. Temperature for sepsis

- **Shock**
  - **Definition**: circulatory failure leading to inadequate organ perfusion.
  - **Remember**: MAP = CO x SVR - shock can be loss or CO or SVR or both
    - Low CO
      - Hypovolemia
        - Bleeding – trauma, ruptured AAA, GI bleed
        - Fluid loss – pancreatitis, heat stroke
      - Pump failure
        - Cardiogenic – ACS, Arrhythmia, Aortic dissection, Acute valve failure
        - Secondary – PE, Tension pneumothorax, Cardiac tamponade
    - Low SVR ("**SANE D**")
      - **S**epsis - Cytokines cause vasodilation. Patients often warm + vasodilated + bounding pulse
      - **A**naphylaxis - Wheeze, stridor, angioedema, urticaria
      - **N**eurogenic - Spinal cord injury, Epidural or spinal anaesthesia

- - **E**ndocrine - Addison's, Hypothyroidism
    - **D**rugs - Anaesthetics, anti-hypertensives, CN poisoning (reduced aerobic respiration)
  - **ABCDE** - the focus is on **Circulation**
    - Cold & clammy - think cardiogenic or hypovolemic shock
    - Warm & well perfused = likely septic or neurogenic shock
    - HR = likely high unless B-blocker or spinal shock
    - BP = narrow pulse pressure with Aortic Stenosis or simply volume depletion
    - BP both arms = dissection if >20mmHg difference
    - Raised JVP = likely cardiogenic
    - Abdominal exam = ?Trauma ? AAA ?GI Bleed
    - **NOTE**: A patient may be initially agitated in SHOCK or ALCOHOL as these affects INHIBITORY areas of the brain first

- **Septic Shock**
  - **Definition**: sepsis with hypotension despite adequate fluid resuscitation OR requiring vasopressors to maintain blood pressure
  - **Presentation**: drowsiness, increased HR, increased RR, increased Lactate, low BP, FEVER
  - **ABCDE** - the focus is on completing your **"Sepsis Six"** - (give 3, take 3)
    - Give 3
      - Oxygen
      - IV broad-spectrum antibiotics with 1 HOUR   `
      - IV fluids
    - Take 3
      - Blood cultures (± urine, sputum, CSF - complete a septic screen)
      - Urine output (by catheterising the patient)
      - Arterial Blood Gas (including Lactate)
  - **Remember**:
    - Refractory SBP<90mmHg OR Lactate >4 → consider early HDU/ ITU referral

33

- You can remember the "Sepsis Six" with "BUFALO" - Bloods, Urine, Fluids, Antibiotics, Lactate, Oxygen

- **Hypovolemic shock**
  - Carry out your ABCDE assessment - Identifying and treating anomalies
  - Raise legs, give fluids (titrated to HR, BP, Urine output), liaise early with seniors regarding escalation (ITU in refractory hypovolemic shock)

- **Haemorrhagic shock**
  - Stop bleeding (depending on the source this may require referral to Gastroenterologists/ Endoscopists [Upper GI bleed] OR Surgeons)
  - Raise legs, give fluids (titrated to HR, BP, Urine output), liaise with seniors regarding escalation
  - Haemorrhage estimated at >30% total blood volume = Activate the **Massive Haemorrhage Protocol -** administering O Rh -ve blood until units are Cross-matched
  - Liaise with seniors/ haematology regarding replacement of Red Bloods Cells: Fresh Frozen Plasma

- **Anaphylaxis**
  - Especially likely with an identifiable TRIGGER - Eg. During blood transfusion/ Contrast imaging/ Medication administration/ Food exposure
  - **Presentation**: Sudden onset of wheezing, Stridor, Angioedema
  - **Management**: "**ROHAS FC**"
    - **Reassure** patient
    - **Oxygen** 15L 100% via NRB
    - **Help** - AIRWAY OF GREAT IMPORTANCE – CALL PERI ARREST TEAM TO SECURE AIRWAY BY INTUBATION
    - **Adrenaline** IM (adult dose 500 mcg = 0.5ml 1:1000 IM in Anterolateral 1/3 of thigh) – repeat every 5 minutes guided by BP, HR, RR
    - **IV** access
    - **Steroid** – Hydrocortisone IV (adult dose 200mg)

- **Fluids** – IV Fluid bolus 500ml 0.9% NaCl over 15 minutes – set up infusion
- **Chlorphenamine** IV (adult dose 10mg)
- Additionally:
    - Consider Nebulised Adrenaline if wheeze
    - Measure Mast Cell Tryptase at 1-6h (confirms anaphylaxis)
    - NOTE: Anaphylaxis implies prior sensitisation IgE mediated Type1 reaction – can test with RAST; Anaphylactoid reaction is different (Common with N-Acetyl Cysteine for treatment of Paracetamol Overdose) No immunoglobulin, simply mast cell degranulation – RAST tests wouldn't show

- **ACS (ST-Elevation Myocardial Infarction)**
    - **Presentation**: Chest pain, SOB, Unexplained syncope (silent MI especially in Diabetics)
    - **ABCDE** - remember:
        - Troponin, D-dimer, BNP
    - **Management**: "**MONARTH**"
        - **Morphine** – 5 mg IV (+ Metoclopramide 10mg IV or 2nd line Cyclizine 50mg IV)
        - **Oxygen** – if sats <94% or SOB
        - **Nitrates** – Sublingual GTN 2 puffs S/L
        - **Aspirin** 300mg PO
        - **Reperfusion** – contact cardiology once ECG carried out – consider referral for primary PCI if (1) present within **12h** of Sx and (2) Possible within **120min of 1st medical contact!** Otherwise **Fibrinolysis** (tPA: Alteplase, tenecteplase – max **24h**; ideal within **30mins** - NOTE: if fibrinolysis, follow-up patient with ECG @90 minutes and if <50% improvement in ST elevation – transfer for rescue PCI
        - **Ticagrelor** – 180 mg PO
        - **Heparin** – UFH or LMWH even if patient for PCI
        - Additionally
            - Criteria for thrombolysis

- ST elevation >1mm in 2+ <u>limb</u> or >2mm in 2+ <u>chest</u>
- **LBBB**
- **Posterior changes – deep ST depression and TALL R in V1-V3**
- **Contra-indications for thrombolysis:** Intracranial haemorrhage, Ischaemic stroke <6 months, GI bleed <1 month, Aortic dissection, Punctures <24h (Ex. Lumbar puncture), major surgery or trauma <3 weeks, known bleeding disorder
  - Following immediate setting - implement secondary prevention: "**ABCES**"
    - **A**spirin
    - **B**-blocker
    - **C**lopidogrel
    - A**CE**-inhibitor
    - **S**tatin
  - Complications you may encounter following STEMI:
    - Recurrent ischaemia or failure to reperfuse – rescue PCI
    - Stroke
    - Cardiogenic shock
    - HF
    - Pericarditis – **Aspirin** (Avoid NSAIDs acutely due to risk impaired scar formation)

- <u>**ACS – Non-ST-Elevation Myocardial Infarction/ Unstable Angina**</u>
  - **Presentation & ABCDE** assessment as above
    - Troponin is especially important to distinguish UA from NSTEMI
  - **Management = "MONARCH"**
    - **Morphine** 10mg IV (+ Metoclopramide 10mg IV or 2nd line Cyclizine 50mg IV)
    - **Oxygen** 15L 100% NRB
    - **Nitrates** – GTN 2 puffs S/L

- **Aspirin** 300mg PO
- **Reperfuse** – depending on GRACE/ TIMI score
- **Clopidogrel** 300mg PO
- **Heparin** or LMWH/ Fondaparinux – continue until discharge
- Additionally, after medical management, calculate GRACE/ TIMI Score to decide whether high risk and need Angiography for PCI or CABG
    - Low risk - treat medically and arrange stress test, angiogram
    - High risk - Infusion of GpIIb/IIIa antagonist (Tirofiban, Ebciximab, Eptifibatide) + refer for Angiography

- <u>**Acute Pulmonary Oedema**</u>
    - Presentation - crackles/wheeze, foamy sputum, increased JBP, high HR, high RR
    - ABCDE - Remember:
        - CXR - may show yet another "ABCDE" (**A**lveolar oedema (Bat's wings)Interstitial oedema (Kerley **B** lines), **C**ardiomegaly, **D**ilated Upper lobe vessels, **E**ffusions – blunted costophrenic angles)
        - ECG (may reveal MI, arrhythmia)
        - Echocardiogram
        - Plasma BNP or pro-BNP
    - Management - "**LMNOP**"
        - **L**oop diuretics - Furosemide 40mg IV – boluses according to hospital protocol
        - DIA**M**orphine [VASODILATORS ARTERIAL SYSTEM] - 1.25mg IV Diamorphine (Beware liver failure, COPD)
        - **N**itrates [VENODILATORS] - GTN spray 2 puffs SL (NOT if SBP<90)
        - **O**xygen - 15L 100% O2 NRB
        - **P**osition - Sit patient upright

- <u>**Broad Complex Tachycardia**</u>
    - **Definition**: ECG rate >100 + QRS >120ms
    - Can be: VT, SVT with BBB, Preexcited tachycardia (AF, AFlutt, AVRT + WPW)
    - **ABCDE** considerations

- Oxygen if sats <94
- CXR
- Cardiac monitor
- IV access
- Correct electrolyte abnormalities (K+ or Mg2+)
- **Management**
  - Pulseless = pulseless VT → Follow Cardiac Arrest ALS algorithm above
  - Are there **adverse signs** (Remember "HISS" - Heart failure, Ischaemia [Chest pain], Shock [SBP<90], Syncope)
    - Yes
      - Immediate DC Cardioversion
      - Call an anaesthetist as this is painful and you will require sedation
    - No → Is QRS regular?
      - Regular
        - VT/ Uncertain rhythm - 300mg IV Amiodarone over 20-60 minutes then 900mg over 24 hours
      - Irregular
        - Seek expert help
        - Could be AF + BBB - try IV Adenosine
        - Polymorphic VT – **IVI MgSO4 2g over 20 minutes**

- <u>**Narrow Complex Tachycardia**</u>
  - **Definition** - ECG = >100bpm BUT QRS <120ms
  - Can be:
    - Sinus tachycardia (Fever, hypovolemia, etc. – if troublesome, rate control w/ B-blocker)
    - Atrial tachyarrhythmia
      - AF = NO P WAVES, IRREGULARLY IRREGULAR QRS
      - A flutter – sawtooth baseline, usually reentrant circuit in RA. Ventricles often at 150 = 2:1

- Atrial tachycardia – abnormally shaped p waves
- Multifocal atrial tachycardia - >3 P wave morphologies
- Junctional tachycardia
  - AVNRT – slow pathway at AVN allows re-entry
  - AVRT – accessory pathway – Ex. Bundle of Kent in WPW
- **Management**
  - Irregular - manage as **AF** – (Rate vs Rhythm = no difference in mortality – difference is only in Symptoms)
    - Stable
      - <48h
        - **Electrical** cardioversion with synchronised DC shock
        - **Pharmacological** cardioversion – Flecainide (no structural abnormality)/ Amiodarone (Structural abnormality)/ Sotalol You can **carry out an ECHO** to check for abnormalities
      - >48
        - If anticoagulated with warfarin for 3 weeks then electrical cardioversion if fine
        - Opt for rate if patient is >65 year old/ has a Hx of IHD → use a B-blocker/ Calcium-Channel Blocker/ Digoxin (especially if co-existent HF)
    - Unstable
      - Heparinise + Sedate + Carry out DC cardioversion
  - Regular
    - Valsalva manoeuvre or carotid sinus massage (transiently increase AV block)

- Adenosine 6mg, 12mg, 12mg (Verapamil if asthma but NOT if on B-b)
- Adverse signs?
  - No – B-blockers, CCb, Digoxin, Amiodarone, Overdrive pacing
  - Yes – Sedation (Midaz) -> Synchronised DC cardioversion -> Amiodarone
- **Wolff-Parkinson-White**
  - Short PR, widened QRS with upstroke DELTA WAVE
  - Management = Flecainide / Amiodarone / Sotalol – refer cardiology for ablation accessory pathway

- <u>**Bradyarrhythmia**</u>
  - **Management**
    - Adverse features? ("HISS" as above)
      - Yes
        - 1st: IV atropine 500mcg
        - 2nd: Consider
          - Repeat IV atropine 500mcg to maximum 3mg
          - Transcutaneous pacing
          - IV Isoprenaline 5mcg/min OR IV Adrenaline 2-10mcg/ min
      - No
        - Risk of asystole? (complete heart block, recent asystole, ventricular pause >3 seconds, Mobitz Type 2 block)
          - Yes
            - As above for (Yes)
          - No
            - Observe

- <u>**Asthma**</u>
  - **Presentation**: Cough, SOB, Wheeze
  - **Classification**
    - Moderate – PEFR 50-70% predicted

- Acute severe – PEFR 33-50% / RR>25 / HR>110 / Unable to complete sentences
- Life threatening – PEFR <33% / Sats <92& / Silent chest / Reduced consciousness / Rising PaCO2 / Falling pH
  - **ABCDE** - extra considerations:
    - Peak Expiratory Flow Rate
  - Management
    - **NB: History of brittle asthma with previous ITU admission = ADMIT REGARDLESS OF SEVERITY**
    - Remember "OSHI(E)M"
      - **O**xygen – 15L 100% NRB
      - **S**albutamol – 5mg NEB (May need to give back-back every 15min à monitor ECG)
      - **H**ydrocortisone – 100mg IV OR Prednisolone 40mg PO
      - **I**pratropium Bromide – 500mcg NEB
      - **E**scalate to consider MgSO4 (2g IV over 20 minutes, Single dose)
      - Acute severe / Life-threatening = warn ICU + SENIORS

- **Chronic Obstructive Pulmonary Disease**
  - Presentation - Cough, SOB, Wheeze
  - **ABCDE** - extra considerations:
    - Peak Expiratory Flow Rate
    - Theophylline levels if on it at home
    - Sputum culture if purulent sputum
    - Blood cultures if fever
  - **Management** - Remember "**OSHI(E)T**"
    - **O**xygen – if very unwell 15L otherwise 24% Venturi – do early ABG
    - **S**albutamol – 5mg NEB
    - **H**ydrocortisone – 100mg IV
    - **I**pratropium Bromide – 500mcg NEB
    - **E**scalate for BiPAP (pH<7.35) OR Intubation & Ventilation (pH<7.25) OR Doxapram (respiratory stimulant)
    - **T**heophylline DECIDED BY SENIORS!
    - Consider antibiotics if sputum purulent

- **Pneumothorax**
  - **Presentation**: acute SOB, pleuritic chest pain
  - Examination: reduced chest expansion, hyperresonant percussion, reduced air entry auscultation
  - **Management**: determined by CXR and symptoms
    - PRIMARY pneumothorax (no underlying lung disease, precipitant)
      - SOB and/ or rim >2cm on CXR?
        - No = SENIOR ADVICE + send home with advice, safety-net; follow-up CXR 2 weekly until recovered
        - Yes = SENIOR ADVICE + aspirate
          - Successful aspiration?
            - No = Chest drain
            - Yes = SENIOR ADVICE + send home with advice
    - SECONDARY pneumothorax (lung disease, trauma, other precipitant)
      - <1cm = Admit 24h for observation
      - 1-2cm / <50 / ASx = Admit + Attempt aspiration
      - 2+cm or Sx = Admit + Chest drain
      NOTE: Chest drain should be removed 24h after lung re-expanded and air leak stopped. This is done during expiration OR valsalva

- **Tension Pneumothorax**
  - **Pathophysiology** - 1 way valve allows air to be sucked in, increases pressure on that side, pushes mediastinum, KINKS great veins, prevents venous return = fall Stroke Volume = fall Cardiac Output
  - **Management**
    - Immediate needle decompression 2nd ICS MCL (now 10th edition ATLS 5th ICS MCL) 14-16G needle partially filled with saline
    - Then inform **SENIORS for CXR + CHEST DRAIN** (blunt dissection in safe triangle)

- **Pneumonia**
    - **Definition**: Infection of lung parenchyma
    - Common organisms: Strep (commonest), Haemophilus (COPD), Mycoplasma (EM, Hemolytic anaemia), Staph (ICU, post influenza), Klebsiella (alcoholics)
    - **ABCDE** extra considerations:
        - Atypical serology
        - Urine - legionella, pneumococcal antigen
        - Bronchoscopy if ?Pneumocystis jirovecii
    - **Severity** according to CURB-65 Score
        - Confusion
        - Urea >7
        - RR >30
        - BP S<90 / D<60
        - Age >65
        0-1 = home, 2 = hospital, 3 = ICU (Also consider ITU if co-existing disease, bilateral or multi lobe involvement, SaO2<92, PO2<8)
    - Management - Remember 3 items
        1. Oxygen
            - 15L 100% NRB
            - If still hypoxic consider CPAP then NIV then Intubation on ITU
        2. Antibiotics
            - Follow local protocol
            - Discuss with microbiology
            - Usually:
                - Community Acquired Pneumonia
                    - Mild = Amoxicillin
                    - Severe = Amoxicillin + another (discuss micro)
                - Hospital Acquired Pneumonia
                    - <5d into admission = Co-amoxiclav
                    - >5d admission = Tazocin
        3. Analgesia
            - Paracetamol/ NSAID for pleuritic pain which may make coughing more difficult

- **Pulmonary Embolism**

- **Presentation** - Acute SOB, pleuritic chest pain, haemoptysis
- **ABCDE** considerations
    - Calculate Well's Score
        - 4 or less = LOW risk à D-dimer
        - 5 or + = High risk à CTPA (IF DELAY >4h in getting scan = LMWH COVER)
- **Management**
    - **Oxygen** – 15L O2 100% NRB
    - **Morphine** IV
    - Start **Warfarin** + **LMWH** and stop when INR 2.5 for >24h or 5 days
        - Target = 2.5 (but 3.5 if recurrence whilst on warfarin)
        - Treatment duration 3 months if provoked, 6 months if unprovoked – then reassess risks + benefits of extending further
        - NOTE: Use
            - LMWH **only** for 6 months in cancer
            - LMWH only for pregnancy
            - Unfractionated Heparin for CKD
            - Lifelong treatment if recurrent PE/ thrombophilia
    - **In massive PE** (haemodynamic compromise) – Urgent senior review for consideration of Thrombolysis – (50mg bolus Alteplase)

    - **Future management** - discuss with Haematology
        - Thrombophilia tests IF
            - No predisposing factors
            - Recurrent DVT
            - FHx DVT
        - Look for underlying malignancy
            - IF PE in patient >40: with Urinalysis, FBC, LFT, Ca2+, CXR
            - Also order CTAP + mammogram if patient is Female

- **Upper Gastrointestinal Bleeding**
  - **Presentation**: Haematemesis, melaena, syncope, signs of hypovolemia/ shock
  - 5 Common causes to consider
    1. PUD
    2. Duodenal erosions/ gastropathy
    3. Oesophagitis
    4. Mallory-weiss tear (will likely stop spontaneously)
    5. Varices
  - **ABCDE** assessment specific considerations:
    - C
      - Obtain IV access x2 large bore cannulae
      - Cross-match
      - Clotting studies
      - LFTs for liver disease
      - Calculate Blatchford score – Urea, Hb, SBP, HR, etc.
    - E
      - Abdominal examination to look for peritonism + inguinal orifices
      - Peripheral oedema/ ascites – cirrhotic patients with variceal bleeds
      - PR exam for melaena
  - **Management**
    - Keep patient nil by mouth + notify surgeons early if severe
    - Bleep Endoscopist – IMMEDIATE if patient is shocked
    - Drug treatment pre-endoscopy
      - PUD = NONE
      - Varices
        - Abx – Cef + Quinolone
        - Terlipressin (OR Octreotide if IHD)
    - IF massive bleed activate major haemorrhage protocol, transfusing ORh-ve blood until Crossmatch
    - Correct clotting abnormalities

  - **Specific management at endoscopy:**
    - Calculate ROCKALL SCORE for prognostication
    - PUD

1. Endoclips
2. Inject dilute Adrenaline
3. Thermal therapy
- Varices
    1. Oesophageal = Banding
    2. Gastric = injection sclerotherapy
    3. 2nd line
        - TIPS + give lactulose to prevent hepatic encephalopathy
        - Sengstaken Blakemore tube to arrest bleed
    - Following successful endoscopic therapy in Ulcer bleed – give PPI IV for 72h infusion
- Check for and eradicate H.pylori in ALL PATIENTS (Triple therapy)

- **Meningitis**
    - **Presentation**: fever, photophobia, phonophobia, neck stiffness
    - **Organisms**: Organisms
        - (Remember "BabyBEL") 0-3m – Group B Strep, E-coli, Listeria
        - (Remember "NHS") 3-6y – Meningococcus, Pneumococcus, Haemophilus
        - 6-60y – Meningococcus, Pneumococcus
        - >60y – Meningococcus, Pneumococcus, Listeria
        - Immunocompromised – Listeria, Cryptococcus, Toxoplasmosis, TB, CMV
    - **ABCDE** specific considerations
        - Glucose
        - Coagulation screen
        - CT then LP – normal pressure = 10-20cmH20
            - Send for MC&S, gram-stain, protein, glucose, virology/PCR, lactate
    - **Management**
        - Cefotaxime 2g IV ± Ampicillin 2d IV (Check local protocol!)
            - Out of hospital - administer IM BenPen
        - IV fluids

- Escalate early - Seniors, ITU, Microbiology, Public Health consultant
    - ITU especially if patient shows signs of shock
- Consider IV Dexamethasone

- **Encephalitis**
    - **Presentation** - like meningitis but with impaired consciousness/ odd behaviour
    - **ABCDE** considerations
        - Blood cultures, viral PCR of serum, malaria film
        - Contrast CT (focal bilateral temporal lobes in HSV encephalitis)
        - Lumbar Puncture - including HSV PCR
    - **Management**
        - Acyclovir within 30 minutes as empirical treatment for Herpes Simplex Virus → administer for 14 days (21 days if immunocompromised)
        - Adjust management liaising with Microbiology
            - CMV - IV Gancyclovir or PO Valganciclovir
            - Toxoplasmosis - Pyrimethamine + Sulfadiazine

- **Status Epilepticus**
    - **Definition**: seizure lasting >5mins OR repeated seizures without consciousness returning in between
    - **Management**
        - Start a clock
        - Don't be afraid to put out an early crash call if you're worried about the patient's airway! It's ALWAYS better to be safe.
        - 0 minutes
            - Regular ABCDE assessment
        - 5 minutes in
            - 1st dose: IV Lorazepam/ PR Diazepam/ Buccal Midazolam
            - Senior review
        - 15 minutes in
            - 2nd dose: IV Lorazepam/ PR Diazepam/ Buccal Midazolam

- Urgent senior review to prepare for next step
  - 25 minutes in
    - IV Phenytoin/ IV Phenobarbital
    - Urgent anaesthetics/ ITU input to prepare for next step
  - 45 minutes in
    - Rapid sequence induction with Sodium Thiopental and EEG monitoring on ITU
  - NOTE: If this occurs in pregnancy - assume Eclampsia - Bleep Obstetrics for delivery of foetus (urinalysis, BP useful in the interim)
  - Remember: During your ABCDE assessment, correct possible causes as they arise - glucose, electrolytes, sepsis, BP abnormalities, alcohol withdrawal, etc.

- **Raised Intracerebral Pressure**
  - **Definition**: volume increase inside the cranium overcomes the ability of CSF/ venous shunting to compensate (Monro-Kellie hypothesis)
  - **Causes**: trauma, space occupying lesion, bleeding, infection, etc.
  - **Presentation**: headache worse on straining/ coughing/ morning, drowsiness/ coma, Cushing's Triad (Remember this as the opposite of what you'd expect in shock - falling HR, falling RR, rising BP), Cheyne-stokes breathing, pupillary dilatation/ papilloedema on fundoscopy
  - **Management**: Remember "**LHOC**" as in "Loss (H) Of Consciousness"
    - **Lie** - elevate the head 30-40° to facilitate venous drainage
    - **Hypotension** - correct low BP to paintain MAP>90 - this may seem nonsensical but remember you must maintain a minimum systemic BP to ensure you retain adequate Cerebral Perfusion Pressure despite a raised Intracranial Pressure
    - **Osmotic agents** - discuss with a senior the use of Mannitol as this can cause an increase in ICP later

- **Corticosteroids** - consider IV dexamethasone in raised ICP due to a suspected tumour or vasculitis process
- Other considerations
    - Early neurosurgical referral for consideration of Craniotomy/ Burr hole → especially important in pre-coning, with Cushing's Triad or Pupillary changes
    - If intubated, consider discussion with a senior regarding Hyperventilation - this causes cerebral vasoconstriction, reducing ICP but will also lead to reduced cerebral perfusion which could aggravate a hypoxic injury

- **Head Injury**
    - **ABCDE considerations:**
        - A patient with a **serious** head injury may require a <u>Trauma Call</u> with input from Emergency Medicine, Anaesthetics, Orthopaedic Surgery, General Surgery and Radiography/ Nursing colleagues
            - For a trauma call, follow C-ABCDE (Excluding Catastrophic Haemorrhage as your first priority)
        - A - remember C-spine 3 point immobilisation and use a jaw thrust as opposed to a head-tilt chin lift if you require airway manoeuvres - liaise with an anaesthetist early on
        - E - palpate the skull for deformity, inspect skull for CSF leak/ Battle's Sign/ Raccoon Eyes/ Haemotympanum on otoscopy → Basal Skull Fracture will require:
            - Neurosurgical referral, CT head, Tetanus status review
    - **CT head criteria**
        - CT head within 1 HOUR
            - GCS <13 on admission
            - GCS <15 at 2 hours
            - Focal neurology
            - Vomiting >once
            - Seizure

- Suspected basal skull #
- CT head within 8 HOURS
  - Anticoagulated patients
  - Amnesia OR Loss of consciousness + 1 of:
    - Patient >65y old
    - Coagulopathy
    - Dangerous mechanism of injury = fall greater than
      - 5 stairs
      - 1 meter
- **CT Spine criteria**
  - GCS <13 on admission
  - Intubation required
  - Pre-operatively (or when urgent diagnosis of C-spine injury needed)
  - Patient undergoing head scan
  - Patient has suspected C-spine injury +1 of:
    - Patient >65y old
    - Paraesthesia
    - Focal CNS deficit
    - Dangerous mechanism of injury

- <u>**Subarachnoid Haemorrhage**</u>
  - **Presentation**: sudden onset thunderclap headache, neck stiffness, consciousness affected, focal neurology, absence of fever
  - **ABCDE** considerations
    - CT/ MRI brain
    - Lumbar puncture - up to 2 weeks, Xanthochromia
  - **Management**
    - (1) Liaise with seniors (2) Urgent Neurosurgical review (3) ICU if falling GCS
    - Lie patient flat
    - Administer appropriate analgesia (Opioids + Anti-emetics)
    - Consider NIMODIPINE (CCB prevents arterial spasm)
    - Dexamethasone if increased ICP

- <u>**Stroke**</u>
  - **ABCDE** considerations

- CT brain
- **Management**
  - Aspirin 300mg PO/PR (after haemorrhagic stroke excluded by imaging)
  - THROMBOLYSIS if:
    - within 4.5h
    - Haemorrhagic stroke excluded
    - No contraindications
  - Additionally:
    - AF? Exclude haemorrhagic stroke and wait 14d after ischaemic stroke before starting patient on Warfarin
    - Cholesterol >3.5 → statin. May delay 48h due to risk haemorrhagic transformation
    - Secondary prevention:
      - Clopidogrel (lifelong) OR aspirin + dipyridamole (lifelong)
      - Carotid endarterectomy if carotid stenosis >70%

- **Aortic Dissection**
  - **Presentation**: Tearing pain
  - **ABCDE** considerations
    - USS/ CT
    - IV access x2 large bore cannulae
    - Antibiotics
    - Analgesia
  - **Management**
    - Immediate referral to (1) vascular surgeons (2) anaesthetist (3) CEPOD
    - Keep SBP <110mmHg with IV Labetalol

- **Severe Hypertension**
  - **Presentation**: continuous throbbing headache, papilloedema on fundoscopy, BP>=180/120 with evidence of acute organ damage
  - **Management**
    - Over days, slowly reduce BP to prevent cerebral infarction by acute reductions in CPP
      - PO Atenolol
      - PO Long-acting CCB

- **Hypertensive encephalopathy or hypertensive congestive cardiac failure** is different:
  - **Management**
    - Admit the patient and insert an intra-arterial line
    - IV therapy is required to lower SBP to 110mmHg over 4 hours (double check hospital protocol)
      - IV Furosemide
      - IV Labetalol
      - IV Sodium Nitroprusside infusion

- <u>Pheochromocytoma</u>
  - **Presentation**: sudden onset fear/ anxiety/ sweating/ headaches/ hypertension
  - **ABCDE** consideration
    - Urinary metanephrine levels
  - **Management**
    - Senior help, may require ITU admission
    - Alpha block 1st **THEN** B-block with LABETALOL as has greater alpha effect than any other B-blocker
      - Alpha-block
        - First short acting – phentolamine
        - Second longer acting – phenoxybenzamine / doxazosin
      - Beta-block
        - Labetalol
    - Surgery
      - After 4-6 weeks – usually adrenalectomy then check response w/ 24h urinary metanephrines (lifelong hormone replacement required)

- <u>Pancreatitis</u>
  - **Presentation** - severe epigastric pain, worse leaning forward, shock
  - **ABCDE** considerations
    - Calculate a modified glasgow score - "**PANCREAS**" - 3+ → consider ITU
      - **P**aO2 <8

- **A**ge >55
- **N**eutrophils >15
- **C**alcium <2
- **R**enal (Urea) >16
- **E**nzymes (LDH) >600 (AST) >200
- **A**lbumin <32
- **S**ugar (Glucose) >11
- Spiral contrast enhanced CT
- **Management**
  - IV FLUIDS - lots of them to counter 3rd space fluid sequestration, titrated to adequate urine output >0.5ml/kg/h
  - Analgesia - Pethidine or morphine
  - Have early threshold for escalation - necrotising pancreatitis/ collection/ ARDS

- <u>**Acute Kidney Injury**</u>
  - **Classification**
    - Pre-renal – hypotension (sepsis, hypovolemia, cardiac)
    - Renal – drugs, GN, vasculitis
    - Post-renal – obstruction
  - **ABCDE** considerations
    - Early ABG/VBG for K+
    - ECG for K+ affecting heart
    - Renal screen bloods
    - Urinalysis
  - **Management** - Remember "Urgent + FLUIDS"
    - **<u>Urgent</u>** escalation to seniors AND nephrologists if:
      - Hyperkalaemia, Pulmonary oedema, uraemic complications, severe metabolic acidosis
    - **F**luid bolus if dehydrated (500ml 0.9% NaCl)
    - **L**ow BP (SBP<110mmHg) - also warrants fluid bolus
    - **U**rinalysis for ALL
    - **I**maging – urgent renal USS if suspected obstruction or no clear cause of AKI identified
    - **D**rugs – Stop nephrotoxic drugs for all (metformin if creatinine rising (risk of lactic acidosis), NSAIDS, nephrotoxic antibiotics (eg

gentamicin, nitrofurantoin), diuretics, ACE-I, ARBs)
- **S**epsis – Sepsis 6 if signs of sepsis

- **Diabetic Ketoacidosis**
  - Low insulin → cannot use glucose → starvation state → ketosis for energy production (Acetone – fruity breath)
  - **Presentation**: polyuria, dehydration, vomiting, abdominal pain (pancreas strain/ ileus from fluid loss/ direct cause of pain by ketones), Kussmaul breathing, anorexia, ketotic breath
  - **Diagnose** triad of:
    1. High glucose – BM>11mmol/L
    2. Ketones – >3mmol/L
    3. Acidaemia – pH<7.3 or Bicarbonate <15
  - **ABCDE** considerations
    - Ketones in blood with capillary ketone strips
  - **Management** - Remember "FIKDH"
    - Fluids - 500ml fluid boluses, consult hospital protocol + discuss with senior/ diabetes team. Continuously reassess and expect to give over 8L over several hours
    - Insulin - Fixed Rate IV Insulin Infusion – 0.1 Units/kg/h [50 units actrapid in 50ml 0.9% NaCl] → This is DOUBLE the dose in HHS (see below)
    - K+ replacement - when urine output adequate, start K+ replacement unless K+ is high. Monitor U&Es every 1 hour
    - Dextrose - Once BM<15 continue insulin to switch off ketogenesis so to prevent causing hypoglycaemia → 10% dextrose infusion alongside NaCl
    - Heparin/ LMWH → prothrombotic state

- **Hyperosmolar Hyperglycemic State (HHS)**
  Hyperglycaemic Hyperosmolar Non-Ketotic Coma (HONK)
  - **Management** - Remember "F(I)KDH"
    - Fluids - 500ml fluid boluses, consult hospital protocol + discuss with senior/ diabetes team
    - (Insulin → ONLY if BM not falling by >5mmol/L/h → use Fixed Rate IV Insulin

Infusion – 0.05 Units/kg/h → This is HALF the dose in DKA)
- K+ replacement - when urine output adequate, start K+ replacement unless K+ is high. Monitor U&Es every 1 hour
- Dextrose
- Heparin/ LMWH → prothrombotic state

- **Hypoglycaemia**
  - **Presentation**: Hunger, sweating, confusion, loss of consciousness, seizures
  - **Management**:
    - Consult hospital hypoglycaemia protocol, but usually:
    - BM <4 + conscious
      - Glucojuice bottles
    - BM <4 + Confused
      - Glucogel in between gums/ cheeks
    - BM<4 + Unconscious
      - IV dextrose 50ml 50%/ IV dextrose 200ml 10%
      - IM glucagon (NOT in alcohol, AN, malnutrition – as these often cause depleted glycogen stores, which is what glucagon relies on)
    - Once conscious – give sugary drinks + a meal

- **Myxoedema Coma**
  - **Presentation**: Fatigue, bradycardia, cold intolerance, hyporeflexia, coma, seizures
  - **ABCDE** considerations
    - Thyroid function tests
    - Cortisol, glucose
  - **Management**
    - Immediately escalate to seniors/ ITU
    - SLOW IV LIOTHYRONINE (T3) – to avoid precipitating IHD
    - HYDROCORTISONE IV – if unsure if could be due to hypopituitarism
    - Supportive: oxygen, fluids, warming as needed

- **Thyrotoxicosis**

- **Presentation**: Agistation, tachycardia, hyperthermia, hyper-reflexia
- **ABCDE** consideration
  - Hyperthyroid = High BM / Hypothyroid = Low BM → since thyroid hormones make body use up insulin faster
- **Management**
  - Immediately escalate to seniors/ ITU
  - Symptom control - Propranolol/ Diltiazem
  - Direct management
    1. Carbimazole PO/ NGT
    2. THEN Lugol's Iodine to block thyroid
    3. Hydrocortisone OR dexamethasone to prevent peripheral conversion of T4→T3 (more potent)
  - No improvement in 24h – consider THYROIDECTOMY

- **Addison's**
  - **Presentation**: sepsis-like presentation with no fever
  - **ABCDE** considerations
    - Blood cortisol + ACTH
  - **Management**
    - IV Hydrocortisone
    - Consider Fludrocortisone if adrenal disease (DISCUSS WITH SENIOR + ENDOCRINE) – only give it when they are steroid replete (longer-term management)
    - IV Dextrose if hypoglycaemic
    - CAUSE – search + treat → Waterhouse-Friderichsen management = IV hydrocortisone + IV Cefotaxime
    - Long-term
      - Short Synachthen tests – to Dx Adrenal Insufficiency
      - Long Synachthen test – 2° = delayed increase in cortisol (Adrenal atrophied) BUT 1° (Addison's) = impaired throughout

- **Hypopituitary coma**

- **ABCDE** considerations
  - Cortisol, Thyroid function tests, BM
  - CT/ MRI pituitary
- **Management**
  - Hydrocortisone 100mg IV / 6h
  - THEN Liothyronine (T3) IV PO or slow IV
  - Surgery if pituitary apoplexy (bleeding into OR impaired blood supply to pituitary)

- **Post-operative bleeding**
  - **ABCDE** considerations
    - Legs up to shift blood centrally
    - Clotting tests
    - Cross-match
    - Catheter + monitor UO
    - Consider imaging - USS/ CT
  - **Management**
    - Early involvement of seniors/ surgeons/ anaesthetist/ CEPOD
    - Review operation notes - estimated blood loss, specific management plan or advice regarding post-operative bleeding?
    - IV fluids
    - In major bleed, transfuse: (1) Packed RBCs (2) Platelets (3) FFP

- **Burns**
  - **Area of burn**:
    - Rule of 9s
    - Lung & Browder chart
    - Palmar surface = 1%
  - **ABCDE** considerations
    - Wear PPE in chemical burns before approaching patient
    - A
      - Always give 100% Oxygen especially with potential for CO/CN poisoning (where SpO2 unreliable)
      - Burnt airways = immediate anaesthetics input for airway protection
    - B

- Reduced chest expansion in chest burns - consider ESCHAROTOMY
- C
    - IV access preferably through non-burnt tissue
    - U&Es + creatinine – especially due to risk of Rhabdomyolysis from burns
    - Check COHb
- E
    - Temperature ("cool burn, warm patient" - warm IV fluids)
    - Check pulses regularly - loss of pulses → ?compartment syndrome = consider fasciotomy
    - Analgesia - opioids + anti-emetics
- **Management**
    - Bleep ICU + get early advice from major burns center and considering transfer) if:
        - Partial thickness burn >10% child, >15% adult
        - Full thickness burn >2% child, >3% adult
        - Burns to perineum, genitals, face, palms, soles, airway
    - Fluid replacement guided by Parkland formula = 4ml x % burn area x kg (7ml if electrical)
        - This gives you the amount of Hartmann's solution to be administered over 24 hours, with 50% in the first 8h and 50% over subsequent 16h
        - Aim urine output >0.5ml/kg/hr (1-2 if electrical burn/ children)

The following scenarios are unlikely to come up. If they do, stick to your ABCDE assessment, refer early and remember some of the unique management we have included below. You won't be required to mention it in your interviews, but you will be showing a good level of knowledge if you do.

- <u>**Heat stroke/ Hyperthermia**</u>
    - Cool the patient with sponging/ fanning & Resuscitate with IV Infusions

- Do this slow, continuously monitor temperature and stop cooling when T° <39

- **HYPOTHERMIA (core, rectal temperature <35")**
  - **Categories**
    - Mild = patient will be shivering
    - Severe = no shivering, drowsiness/ coma, slow HR, low BP, arrhythmias
  - Monitor temperature with infra-red ear thermometer
  - **Management**
    - Warm the patient with:
      - humidified oxygen
      - warm IV infusion
      - Blankets
      - Bair hugger (hot air duvet)
    - Rewarm 0.5°C/h – monitoring BP, HR, RR – TOO QUICK = VASODILATATION + SHOCK
    - Exception is with sudden (submersion) or profound (<30°) hypothermia → warm rapidly with fluid lavage (Bladder, Nasogastric, Intraperitoneal fluid) or ECMO (intravascular warming)
    - Remember:
      - "A patient is not dead until they are warm and dead" - continue resuscitation for extended periods of time in hypothermia
      - antibiotics to prevent subsequent pneumonia

- **Hyperkalaemia**
  - Emergency = K+ >6 or >5.5 with ECG changes
  - **ECG** - small P, slurred QRS, long PR, tented T
  - **Management**:
    1. Cardiac protection - 10ml 10% Calcium Chloride/ Gluconate
    2. Shift K+ into cells - Salbutamol + Insulin/ Dextrose infusion
    3. Remove K+ from body - Loop diuretics + Calcium resonium PO or ENEMA – takes around 48h + Consider Renal replacement therapy

- **Hypokalaemia**
    - **ECG** - Remember: "No Pot and no T, But a long PR and long QT/ depressed ST" = No Potassium and no T waves but a long PR interval/ QT interval/ depressed ST segment
    - **Management**
        - Mild - PO Potassium (Sando-K)
        - Severe - IV Potassium - maximum 10 mmol/h

- **Hypernatraemia**
    - **Management**
        - Mild - Encourage oral water intake
        - Severe - IV 5% dextrose

- **Hyponatraemia**
    - **Management**
        - Mild - fluid restrict patient
        - Acute - demeclocycline (ADH antagonist) or Vaptans (Vasopressor receptor antagonists)
        - Emergency - hypertonic saline + furosemide (beware HF/ Central pontine myelinolysis)

- **Hypercalcaemia**
    - In Hyperparathyroidism, Sarcoidosis, Multiple myeloma, etc.
    - **Management**
        - IV fluids
        - Bisphosphonates
        - Calcitonin

- **Hypocalcaemia**
    - **Management**
        - Mild = PO Calcium
        - Severe = IV Calcium

- **Hyperphosphataemia**
    - With Chronic Kidney Disease
    - **Management**
        - Calcium carbonate/ Sevelamer (Phosphate binders)

- **Hypophosphataemia**
  - With refeeding syndrome
  - **Management**
    - IV Phosphate

- **Acute Limb**
  - **Management**
    - Call senior help
    - Dependent on suspected diagnosis
      - **Acute ischaemia** – O2, Analgesia, Heparin, Vascular surgeons
      - **Compartment syndrome** – O2, Remove plaster, Orthopaedics
      - **Septic arthritis** – O2, Joint aspiration (except if prosthetic), Orthopaedics
      - **NecFasc** – O2, IV Antibiotics, Surgeons (Type 2 = GAS – BenPen / Type 1 = Mixed – BenPen, Vanc, Met)
      - **Gangrene** – O2, Fluids, IV Antibiotics, Surgeons

- **Aggression**
  - **Management** = Take rational approach
    - Ensure other patients/ staff are safe
    - Ensure your own safety: Is it safe to approach?
      - Yes
        - Try to calm them down
        - Call relatives to help if possible
        - Offer help
        - Reorientate them if they could be delirious
      - No
        - Call senior help + security
    - NOTE: As an F1 you will **not** be sedating a patient with IM Haloperidol or Lorazepam! - don't suggest this in an interview

- **Acute Angle Closure Glaucoma**
  - Management
    - Urgent ophthalmology review
    - Lie the patient flat to encourage the lens to move posteriorly

- Consider Pilocarpine
- Consider Acetazolamide

- **Acute Cauda Equina**
  - **Management**
    - Urgent neurosurgical review
    - Possible malignancy = Dexamethasone IV whilst considering Radiotherapy, Chemotherapy, Decompressive laminectomy
    - Possible abscess = IV Antibiotics + neurosurgical drainage

- **Myasthenic crisis**
  - **Management**
    - Monitor Forced Vital Capacity (<20ml/kg = EMERGENCY - you need an anaesthetist to intubate and ventilate the patient in ITU)
    - Plasmapheresis
    - IV Immunoglobulins

- **Eclampsia**
  - **Management**
    - Urgent referral to Obstetrics for delivery of baby AND PLACENTA
    - CTG monitoring
    - BP control with PO Labetalol
    - Liaise with seniors

- **Acute Psychosis**
  - **Investigation**
    - Patient notes - previous diagnosis of schizophrenia/ Bipolar affective disorder?
    - Organic causes of psychosis - drug screen, CT head, Thyroid function tests, Collateral history from family members, full ABCDE, History and Examination
    - Risk assessment - is the patient a risk to themselves/ others? Will you need to escalate to a senior urgently or call security?
  - **Management**
    - **Mental health condition**

- - Mental Health Act - for doctors this is Section 5(2)
  - **Organic condition/ Temporary impairment of brain function**
    - Mental Capacity Act
    - Discuss with a senior whether you can prevent the patient from self-discharging
    - Consider providing treatment in best interests under **COMMON LAW**
  - **Moving forward**
    - Refer to psychiatry
      - Schizophrenia - Atypical Antipsychotic + Cognitive Behavioural Therapy + Cardiovascular Risk Assessment (due to antipsychotic)
      - BPAD - Mood stabiliser

- **<u>Overdose/ Poisoning</u>**
  - **ABCDE** considerations
    - Use TICTAC system to identify pills if present
    - Discuss overdose with Toxicology services - seek senior advice
    - A
    - B
      - RR<8 / PO2<8 / GCS<8 → ICU / Anaesthetist for airway protection
    - C
      - Toxicology screen - urine and serum
  - **Management**
    - Liaise with seniors and consider
      - Gastric lavage
      - Activated charcoal
      - Haemofiltration
      - Specific antidotes
        - **CO** - 100% oxygen, Hyperbaric O2
        - **Digoxin** - Digibind, Potassium correction
        - **Iron** - desferrioxamine
        - **TCA** - IV lipid emulsion/ IV bicarbonate

- **Benzodiazepines** - IV Flumazenil
- **B-blockers** - IV Atropine, IV glucagon/ dextrose, Cardiac pacing
- **Cyanide** - 100% oxygen/ Sodium thiosulfate/ Sodium nitrite/ Hydroxocobalamin
- **Warfarin**
  - <5 = withhold warfarin
  - 5-8 + No bleed = withhold warfarin 1-2 doses
  - 5-8 + Minor bleed = Stop warfarin + Vit K
  - >8 + No bleed = Stop warfarin + Vit K
  - >8 + Minor bleed = Stop warfarin + Vik K
  - MAJOR bleed = Stop warfarin + Vit K + PCC (Beriplex)
- **Phenothiazines**
  - IV Procyclidine
- **Organophosphates**
  - Witness PNS overdrive: "SLUDGEM" - Salivation, Lacrimation, Urination, Diarrhoea, Emesis, Miosis
  - IV Atropine, IV pralidoxime
- **Cocaine/ Ecstasy**
  - Witness SNS overdrive: overheating, mydriasis
  - Diazepam / Dantrolene / Nifedipine or Phentolamine
- **Salicylate**
  - Activated charcoal <1h
  - Senior advice for:
    - Sodium Bicarbonate

- - Urinary alkalinisation
    - Dialysis
  - **Paracetamol**
    - Activated charcoal <1h
    - N-acetylcysteine
      - <4h = wait until 4h to do levels
      - 4-8h = do levels and start NAC if over treatment line
      - Immediate NAC if overdose is staggered, uncertain time, >8h since presentation – THEN LEVELS and stop if below line
    - Note with NAC: a rash is fine don't stop NAC, only stop if anaphylaxis
    - Consider transfer to liver unit if meeting King's College Hospital criteria of:
      - pH<7.3
      - OR all 3 of:
        - PT>100s
        - SCr>300micro mol/L
        - Grade ¾ encephalopath y
  - Psychiatry review if possible suicide attempt

Chapter 4 – Critical Appraisal Station

Introduction

The key difference between an academic foundation post and a regular clinical post is the dedicated academic time outside of your clinical commitments. It therefore follows that you'll be required to demonstrate your academic capability and aspirations by means of a critical appraisal station. In this section, we'll discuss what you can expect from critical appraisal stations and how to best tackle them.

On interview day, after you've checked in you'll be given two information resources approximately 30 minutes before your interview begins, one for the clinical station and the other for the critical appraisal section. You can expect the latter to be a carefully selected abstract of an academic paper, old or new. You'd be expected to familiarise yourself with this abstract, understand its aim and be ready to critically appraise it in front of a panel of interviewers. Processing a single research abstract does not sound particularly difficult, but under time pressure, being in a new environment, juggling a clinical scenario, impressing the panel and attempting to exceed your talented peers to rank highly in this station is no walk in the park.

If you're wondering who's going to be on your panel to settle your pre-interview anxiety, unfortunately this information will not be made available to you. However, it wouldn't be a bad guess to expect a clinician, non-clinical researcher, academic clinician or someone who is intimately involved with the oversight of foundation doctor roles.

The purpose of this station is to get a narrow insight into your academic capabilities by testing you on your own two feet. The critical appraisal station is one of the few (or perhaps only) chances to impress your interviewers academically and show them that you're more deserving of the post than your competition. Amongst other things, your interviewers will be looking for a general understanding of key academic concepts and an ability to succinctly present and deconstruct an abstract, assessing the scientific validity along the way.

In order to ace the critical appraisal station, a few things will be required of you:

> 1. Prerequisite knowledge of core/advanced academic concepts and definitions.

2. A framework to critically appraise abstracts and a framework to present your thoughts.

3. Plenty of practice with peers/seniors who can provide honest, constructive feedback.

A holistic understanding of academic concepts/definitions is essential if you wish to hit the ground running with your appraisal practice. If you're a bit rusty with common terms (and completely new to others), we've gone ahead and made a whole glossary of definitions to bring you up to speed. It's worth brushing over these before moving on to our abstract appraisal framework and worked examples.

4.1 - Academic Glossary

Types of studies

The following study types (evaluated in more detail below) can be arranged into a well-known 'pyramid/hierarchy of evidence':

1. Systematic reviews and meta-analyses
2. Randomised Controlled Trials (RCTs)
3. Cohort studies
4. Case-control studies
5. Cross-sectional surveys
6. Case-reports

Systematic review ± meta-analysis - A systematic review is a qualitative or quantitative review of all the literature regarding a research question of interest, using a comprehensive search strategy. A systematic review may follow: Preferred Reporting Items for Systematic Reviews and Meta-Analyses ('PRISMA' guidelines [1]- no need to memorise these, but be aware of) guidelines. These include having a clearly defined set of inclusion/exclusion criteria and quality assessing studies before being left with a final batch of studies for review. If the studies have 'homogenous' (similar) study designs and a comparable numerical outcome, statistical analyses can be performed to calculate a total mean effect from the outcomes of all the studies included. E.g. *100 similar studies investigating the effect of drug X on blood pressure were reviewed, a meta-analysis showed that the overall effect from all these studies was a reduction of 10mmHg systolic blood pressure.* If a statistical calculation like this can be calculated, it should be. If it *has* been calculated, this study is now said to be/include a meta-analysis, with a characteristic 'forest plot'* often used to display the individual studies and overall effect size. ***Forest plot (see examples online) -** A plot used in meta-analyses that shows the effect/outcome of each individual study, along with a combined 'overall' outcome. On the x-axis is the study outcome measure (odds ratio, relative risk etc.) Each individual study outcome is plotted as a square (the size of the square corresponds to the size of the study) and two equal lines either side of it (the confidence intervals). The overall combination of all the outcomes is represented as a diamond. The middle of the diamond is the mean value, with the edges corresponding to the confidence interval limits. If any part of the diamond crosses the line of null effect (e.g. if the outcome of interest is odds ratio, the line of null effect will be an odds ratio of 1), it is said there is no significant difference between the treatment of interest and the control.

- Pros: Comprehensive review of all the (high-quality) literature available, permitting a clearer estimate of overall pooled effect size if meta-analyses are performed; resolves uncertainty over conflicting studies; establishes questions for future RCTs/other studies to fill gaps in literature.
- Cons: Subject to publication bias (where certain studies are not published for various reasons - can be highlighted using a 'funnel plot'); selection of studies may introduce bias; heterogeneity of studies and poor methodological quality of selected studies can influence overall effect size/conclusions.

Randomised controlled trial (RCT) - An RCT is a *trial* of a new treatment where recruited patients are *randomised* to either an 'intervention group' (containing the new treatment) or a 'control' group (containing a placebo or similar treatment for comparison). The term *'controlled'* means that everything in the trial apart from the treatment should ideally remain the same. This is to ensure that any observed difference in outcomes is due to the treatment itself as opposed to 'confounding' variables (see confounding variable). RCTs are the highest level of 'primary' evidence (as compared to secondary research - literature/systematic reviews) in the evidence pyramid. A popular set of recommendations for RCT reporting is the Consolidated Standards of Reporting Guidelines (**'CONSORT'** guidelines [2] - no need to memorise them, but to be aware of).

- Pros: Blinding possible; randomisation reduces systematic bias through distribution of confounding factors; evaluation of a single variable; prospective design.
- Cons: Very expensive (funded by bodies with a vested interest?); time-consuming; ethical issues arise if one group deemed to potentially receive weaker treatment or have worse outcomes.

Cohort study - A cohort of people who share a common characteristic are followed up for repeated observations over a period of time (making this a type of longitudinal study) to establish whether this characteristic causes an outcome of interest. This is to establish or refute a 'cause and effect' relationship. The cohort must not already have the outcome of interest at the start of the study. A cohort study design is fundamental in epidemiological studies.

- Pros: Help to identify causality, helps to identify rates of disease and risk, incidence etc. Good for rare exposures/'causes', can help to identify multiple outcomes for given exposure.

- Cons: Can be a lot of people to follow up for a long period of time, expensive, time-consuming, not good for rare diseases, loss to followup introduces bias.

Case-control study - A case-control study is a retrospective analysis of what could have caused an outcome of interest in patients, through comparison of people without the outcome from the same population. E.g. *3 people in a small town have a rare type of cancer (cases), they were compared with other people in the same town population without that cancer (controls), to see what may have caused the cancer in the 'cases' group or protected from cancer in the 'control' group.* This type of study is often used for identifying potential causes of rare diseases, where a large prospective cohort study may not even yield one patient with the disease of interest. The main outcome measure used in these studies is an 'odds ratio' (see Odds Ratio), as 'relative risk' (see Relative Risk) cannot be calculated retrospectively.

- Pros: Quick and inexpensive; relatively few participants required; can be used to evaluate multiple exposures per outcome.
- Cons: Subject to 'recall bias'; difficult to validate information from participants; difficult to select similar; suitable control group.

Cross-sectional study - A snapshot (cross-section) of the characteristics of a population. It can be used to calculate things like prevalence, and understand what is happening in a current population.

- Pros: Quick and inexpensive; allow for analysis of multiple variables;
- Cons: Cannot identify causal relationships; cohort differences (e.g. a snapshot of a population with prevalent asbestosis will not be representative of a later generation who have not been affected); only effective when representative of a whole population; surveys and data collection subject to recall bias

Case-report or case-series - A descriptive story of a single case presentation (often rare or unexpected), highlighting the entire timeframe of events and investigations/decisions carried out by the medical team. Traditionally seen as the weakest form of evidence, these studies can still be crucial for the early warning of unique presentations, detection of previously unknown conditions and alerting clinicians to possible links between exposure and outcome

- Pros: Extremely quick to write up and publish; cheap; informs clinicians about unknown or rare presentations.

- Cons: Plenty of bias; weak evidence.

Common academic terms

P-value - The probability that the null hypothesis is true. Most papers will aim for a P-value of <0.05 (5%) or <0.01 (1%).

> Layman's terms: The p-value is the probability (between 0 and 1, 1 being the highest) that the outcome of an experiment was due to pure chance as opposed to an actual difference.

> Worked example: We want to see if drug X is better than drug Y. The null hypothesis is that both drugs are equally as effective. Our 'alternative' hypothesis is that drug X is better than drug Y. Therefore, we need to carry out an experiment that shows a 'statistically significant' difference of drug X being better, in order to reject the null hypothesis and accept our alternative hypothesis. Our experiment shows that drug X was twice as good as drug Y. The P-value was 0.0001, this is really small and means that the probability of this result being down to chance of our sample is insignificant (i.e. our findings are statistically significant). In other words, the probability that the null hypothesis is actually true despite our result is 0.0001. Most papers will state that any P-value of <0.05 or <0.01 are what they will consider as statistically significant.

Power -The likelihood of a study detecting a true difference. This involves a calculation that determines what sample size will be needed to say a detected outcome is statistically significant when it is in fact significant. I.e. *Reversely, some studies conclude that there was no statistically significant result because they used too small a sample size to detect a significant difference. If in reality, there should have been a statistically significant difference, this study has made a type 2 error (see type 2 error).*

Confidence Interval (CI) - The confidence interval is the range in which you are 95% sure that the real population result lies somewhere between.

> Layman's terms: With any experiment, a sample size can never truly be representative of the wider population (unless your sample is in fact the entire population of interest!). Therefore, the result of any test on a sample cannot be extrapolated to the true population without some sort of statistical guarantee; a 'confidence level'

provides exactly that. Most studies that follow the 'CONSORT' guidelines now include confidence intervals routinely.

Worked example: In our test sample, drug X was 10% more effective than drug Y (95% CI +5 +15). Within the brackets, we have highlighted that we can be (statistically) 95% confident that the true population value of drug X's effectiveness is between 5% and 15% better than drug Y. Conversely, we can only be 5% confident that the true value lies outside of these perimeters (less than 5% or greater than 15%). If our CI was something like '95% CI -5 +25' this would now mean that our CI crosses 0 and even goes into the negative. This tells us that there's a good chance that, in the true population, drug X might actually be less effective (by up to 5%) than drug Y. Moreover, the former CI would be statistically significant and provide a 'definitive' positive result whereas whilst the latter example would provide a 'non-definitive' positive result.

For the next four terms, we'll be referring to example 1 below. It's vital that you familiarise yourself with this example as it represents the simplest method of breaking down some of the key findings of a trial with an intervention and control group.

In the table below, 'events' and 'non-events' refer to the outcome of interest occurring or not occurring. This could be 'dead' or 'alive' after a certain number of years OR 'heart attack' or 'no heart attack' over a period of time etc. A great way to conceptualise the term 'risk' in the following examples is to replace it with the word 'probability', they mean the same thing!

Example 1:

	Group	
	Intervention	Control
Events	A	X
Non-events	B	Y

Absolute Risk (AR) - The probability of an event (or non-event) occurring within a specific group.

In the intervention group for example, the AR of an 'event' occurring is A/A+B. The AR of a 'non-event' occurring is B/A+B. Absolute risks (like probabilities) can only be between the values: 0-1

Absolute Risk Difference/Increase/Reduction - The difference in ARs of an event/non-event in the intervention group compared with the control group.

Think about it like this: did the intervention group reduce the probability ('Absolute Risk') of an 'event' occurring compared with the control group? If so, there was an Absolute Risk *Reduction*. If the probability ('Absolute Risk') of that event increased in the intervention group compared with the control group, there was an Absolute Risk *Increase*.

Relative Risk Reduction/Increase - The absolute risk of an 'event' occurring in the Intervention group compared with the absolute risk of the same event occurring in the Control group.

The probability of an 'event' occurring in the intervention group as a difference from the probability of that same 'event' occurring in the control group. This can be calculated as the following: 1 - (A/A+B $\div$ X/X+Y). Once again, this is only a Relative Risk *Reduction* if the Absolute Risk in question was less in the intervention group than the control group. This value can also be expressed as a percentage.

Number Needed to Treat (NNT) - The number of people needed to treat with the 'intervention' to save *one* person from a bad 'event'.

This is calculated as the inverse of the Absolute Risk *Reduction* (1/ARR).

N.B. If there is an Absolute Risk *Increase*, the inverse of this would provide the '**Number Needed to Harm**'.

Let's now use a simple example as a case study to apply the above terms.

Example 2 - 2000 people with high blood pressure are split equally into 2 groups, one receiving a new drug to lower blood pressure, the other receiving a placebo. They are followed up at 10 years to see which group was more likely to have had at least 1 heart attack.

	Group	
	New Drug	Control
Heart attack	300	400
No heart attack	700	600

Absolute Risk of a heart attack: New drug = 0.3; Control = **0.4**

Absolute Risk Reduction of a heart attack (in 'new drug' group compared with 'control'): **0.1**

Relative Risk Reduction: 1 - (0.3 $\div$ 0.4) = **0.25** or **25%**

Number Needed to Treat: 1 $\div$ 0.1 = **10**

Odds ratio - The odds of an outcome occurring if exposed to something, compared to the odds of that outcome occurring if unexposed to that same thing. Odds does not equal probability; where probability means the fraction of times you expect to see an event occur (between 0-1), odds is the probability of the event occurring divided by the probability of the event not occurring. Odds ratio is often used in case-control studies.

Hazard ratio - At a specific point in time, the probability of an event (often a negative outcome) occurring in the intervention group compared with (divided by) the same probability of that event occurring in the control group. I.e. *In a study, if the hazard ratio of having a stroke is '0.5' (e.g. 1 in 10 divided by 1 in 5) after one year in a study, this means that the intervention group is 50% less likely to have a stroke than the control group at that point in time. A hazard ratio of 3 would mean that the intervention group are 3 times as likely to experience that hazard (compared to the control group) at that point in time.* N.B. This is almost the exact same as relative risk, although this term includes the element of time.

Kaplan-meier curve (search examples online) - This is a graph that shows a 'time to event' analysis, with the event often being death or an alternative ('surrogate') clinical endpoint. In the former case, this may be referred to as a plot of 'survival analysis', commonly used in clinical trial studies looking at the fraction of subjects who are still alive following a treatment, over X amount of time. The plot appears to follow a trend of downgoing steps, with each step corresponding to an 'event' occurring. Along the x-axis is the timeframe, with the final 'step' occurring in conjunction with the final recorded event. Along the graph, a small indicator (usually marked | or +) correlates to the time at which a patient has withdrawn from the study (or follow-up lost), or if the trial itself had finished at that stage of their follow-up. These are known as 'censored events'. It's worth familiarising yourself with these graphs, as you're likely to see them in randomised controlled trials.

Blinding - If participants of a study are blinded to their treatment allocation (intervention vs control), this is known as a '**single blind**' study. If the experimenters allocating treatment, measuring data and analysing it (etc.) are blind to the group allocation, this is said to make the study '**double blind**'. Blinding is an attempt at eliminating bias by the experimenters and participants being aware of the allocated treatment. Intervention and control treatment are often made to be similar in every way apart from the active treatment (e.g. yellow pill containing antibiotic vs identical yellow pill containing non-active substance). In some situations where treatment and control cannot be made identical, a '**double dummy**' design can be used. For example, if a pill is to be compared to a patch, group A may receive the active pill with a placebo patch, group B will receive a placebo pill with the active patch. In this way, both groups take a placebo of some sort.

Confounding variables/factors - A variable/factor that affects the dependent variable but is unaccounted for. This can be reduced by randomisation, blinding and matching groups as best as possible to align baseline characteristics.

Intention-to-treat analysis (ITT) - Analysis of trial participants as per the group they were originally allocated to (irrespective of whether they were non-compliant, withdrew from the study etc.).

Per Protocol analysis (PP) - Analysis of trial participants with exclusion of those who did not follow protocol (non-compliance/withdrew from study etc.). This is to identify the treatment effect under optimal conditions.

Internal validity - The trustworthiness of a study which is seeking to establish a 'cause and effect' relationship, earned through robust methodology and elimination of systematic error/bias. I.e. *If a study has taken appropriate steps to ensure that its findings are not caused incidentally by confounding factors, we can safely say its results and conclusions are internally valid.*

External validity - This is the validity (or generalisability) of the study in the context of the wider population. E.g. *In a study looking at drug X's effect on diabetic outcomes in an south-asian population, the study may have earned the right to be deemed internally valid (lack of systematic bias, robust methodology, valid conclusions etc.), but this study will likely not be generalisable to all ethnicities and populations.* Generalisability is incredibly important when developing new treatments, although studies often may not explicitly highlight their study's drawbacks when it comes to this. A study's exclusion criteria for patients may be a good start for evaluating external validity. I.e. *If a study is evaluating drug Y's efficacy on improving eczema symptoms, excluding patients with severe eczema from the study will mean that this study is not generalisable to them!*

True positive result - Test = positive result. Reality = positive. E.g. A blood test that detects a disease in a person who actually has that disease.

False positive result - Test = positive result. Reality = negative. E.g. A blood test that detects a disease in a person who does *not* have that disease.

True negative result - Test = negative result. Reality = negative. E.g. A blood test that doesn't detect a disease in a person who doesn't have that disease.

False negative result - Test = negative result. Reality = positive. E.g. A blood test that doesn't detect a disease in a person who actually has that disease.

Sensitivity - How good is the test at picking up those who truly have the condition? Calculated as per grid below: $(A \div (A + C)) \times 100$

Specificity - How good is the test at excluding those who do not actually have the condition? Calculated as per grid below: $(D \div (D + B)) \times 100$

Positive Predictive Value (PPV) - Following a positive test, what is the probability that the subject truly has the condition? Calculated as per grid below: $(A \div (A + B)) \times 100$

Negative Predictive Value (NPV) - Following a negative test, what is the probability that the subject does not actually have the condition? Calculated as per grid below: $(D \div (D + C)) \times 100$

N.B: The 'negative' or 'positive' when referring to a result always refers to the outcome of the **test**. The 'true' or 'false' refers to whether this is in agreement/disagreement with the reality (as decided by the current gold standard test).

All above terms are best calculated/visualised using this 2x2 grid to evaluate any diagnostic test:

	Disease +ve	Disease -ve
Test +ve	True positive (A)	False positive (B)
Test -ve	False negative (C)	True negative (D)

Type 1 error - Rejecting the null hypothesis when it is in fact true. I.e. If a researcher generates a statistically significant 'false positive' result, they have made a type 1 error. (see 'false positive result')

Type 2 error - Accepting the null hypothesis when it is in fact false. I.e. If a researcher generates a statistically significant 'false negative' result, they have made a type 2 error. (see 'false negative result')

Types of bias

Sampling/Selection/Allocation bias - When the process of selecting a study sample includes an inherent bias, creating a sample non-representative of the true population of interest. When certain groups or attributes are omitted from the sample, this is called omission bias. When certain groups of people are selected preferentially or for convenience, this is inclusive bias.

Publication bias - A bias introduced when studies that don't attain a significant (or desired) outcome are not published. This particularly affects meta-analyses and can be highlighted using a 'funnel plot' graph. A **funnel plot (see online)** is a scattergraph that can explore the publication bias of a given topic, with the 'effect size' of the study on the x-axis and 'size of the study' on the y-axis. This creates a funnel shape that displays publication bias through empty areas of the funnel, more often due to small studies which fail to show a significant outcome and decide against publishing their results.

Attrition bias - The result of patients who share certain characteristics (e.g. non-compliance, severe adverse effects etc.) withdrawing from a study and consequently skewing the resulting outcomes.

Measurement bias - A bias caused by errors that arise through data collection. For example, if participants recall information incorrectly for a study, this is **recall bias**. If the study involves participants self-enrolling into a survey, this can introduce a **response/non-response bias** (for example, only healthy, medication-compliant individuals enrolling into the survey). **Observer/experimenter bias** is when the outcome assessor is unblinded and 'sees what he/she wants to see' regarding the outcomes of different groups. **Hawthorne effect** - The effect of participants acting differently because they know that they are being observed.

References:

1. Moher D, Liberati A, Tetzlaff J, Altman DG, The PRISMA Group (2009). Preferred Reporting Items for Systematic Reviews and Meta-Analyses: The PRISMA Statement. PLoS Med 6(7): e1000097. doi:10.1371/journal.pmed1000097
2. Schulz KF, Altman DG, Moher D, for the CONSORT Group. CONSORT 2010 Statement: updated guidelines for reporting parallel group randomised trials. BMC Medicine 2010, 8:18. (24 March 2010)

Further reading:

If you want more information about types of bias, the following website is a comprehensive online catalogue that is regularly updated:
https://catalogofbias.org/biases/

NICE glossary: https://www.nice.org.uk/Glossary

Another great resource that we'd recommend if you can afford the time, is: 'How to read a paper - Trisha Greenhalgh', as recommended by a large number of our contributors (see chapter 6).

4.2 - The Critical Appraisal

Critically appraising a research paper is about asking a series of simple but systematic questions exploring the intention of the study, methodological quality, transparency and validity of results and subsequent conclusions. Given enough time and resources, digging into a research paper and highlighting its shortcomings is far from an academic challenge. In the AFP academic station, you'll be expected to appraise a study solely from the abstract of the research paper. In addition, you'll be limited to just 30 minutes (including time taken to consider the clinical emergency resource) to gather your thoughts before being expected to succinctly summarise them to a panel of interviewers.

In order to ensure a timely and systematic appraisal of any abstract, we believe that the gold standard approach to this station is to have a framework, both for the appraisal and the presentation. This will allow you jump into motion the moment the abstract is handed to you, wasting no time in developing an ad-hoc plan and maximising time for critical thinking. Similarly, a framework for summarising a research abstract and its appraisal is key to ensuring a slick and timely presentation.

As with all interviews that are (to an extent) transparent with the contents of each station (combined with corroboration from previous applicants), it's worthwhile familiarising yourself with what is likely to come up to ensure your efforts are spent only in high-yield preparation. For example, the majority of abstracts chosen across various AUoAs are relatively new randomised controlled trial studies from high-impact factor journals. It would therefore be logical (if applying to one of these AUoAs) to spend most of your time practicing the appraisal of RCTs, dedicating a fraction of the time on other types of studies (i.e. systematic reviews, cohort studies etc.).

There are countless resources available to help you structure your thoughts when appraising a research paper. However, very few are designed to compliment a similar format to that of the AFP appraisal station. It therefore follows that one would otherwise have to learn how to critically appraise in a short timeframe alongside formulating a unique and effective framework.

In this section, we've distilled the gold-standard questions for appraising any type of study from a wide variety of validated and respected resources (referenced at the end of this section). From this, we've formulated a unique, high-yield and complete framework for you to apply to all research abstracts henceforth; both for the AFP interview and the future, this framework is easy to follow yet extensive enough for you to take through to higher academic training. For this framework, we've built upon a skeleton that you're probably already familiar with and sure to never forget: the headings of an abstract.

Just so we're on the same page, a typical abstract will look something like this:

TITLE (± AUTHORS)

INTRODUCTION or AIMS or OBJECTIVES or BACKGROUND

METHODS

RESULTS

CONCLUSIONS or DISCUSSION

As you read through an abstract, using each heading as a signpost for necessary questions of appraisal is a sure way to cover all grounds. Below is a full expansion of all the questions you should consider as you begin to read through a research abstract (not exactly applicable to secondary research such as literature/systematic reviews). To keep this section as precise as possible, we haven't expanded on all the sub-questions in detail; to see them applied with context, see the worked examples further down. Notably, not all the questions below can be answered from the small snippet that is the abstract, but, even then, you may still be pushed to consider their answers during your interview.

The 15-minute Abstract Appraisal Framework

Title & Introduction/Aims/Objectives/Background

1. What is the paper about?
   - What is the type of study? (Randomised control trial, cohort study, cross-sectional study, case-control study, systematic review, etc.)
   - What is the research question? Is it a valid question? Is there a clearly defined hypothesis? Are they adding something new/being more rigorous/ larger study? If not, why is this study needed?
   - Are primary/secondary outcomes identified? Are they appropriate?
   - If available, who are the authors and the funders of this study, what are their intentions? Is there an obvious conflict of interest? - Ex. study funded by a drug company that will profit from the sale of the drug

Methods

2. Whom is the study about?
   - What was the inclusion criteria for the study? Was there any recruitment bias?
   - What was the exclusion criteria for the study? Does this make the sample generalisable to the wider population?
   - What was the size of sample? Was this adequately powered?
   - Were participants followed up for an appropriate length of time?
3. Was the study well designed?
   - What intervention was considered?
   - Was there a control? Was this a placebo or current gold standard treatment and was this suitable?
   - What outcome was being measured? Was this sensible and a validated measure for the outcome of interest?
4. How was systematic bias avoided?
   - Were participants randomised? If yes, how? Were baseline characteristics accounted for? If not, are there confounding variables?
   - Were participants blinded? If so, were investigators also blind (double-blind)? Was this done well? Were any biases introduced?

5.   What statistical analyses were carried out? (we know, a bit advanced at this stage)
- o   Were these appropriate? What comparisons were made?
- o   Were the correct statistical tests chosen?

Results

6.   What were the results?
- o   Are the results for all outcomes of interest displayed clearly, even those which don't support the hypothesis?
- o   Were the results statistically significant? What were the confidence limits? Mean? Standard deviation?
7.   Was there loss of follow-up?
- o   How many people withdrew from the trial/study? Is this information clearly available? Could this introduce an attrition bias?
- o   Were results analysed and reported as per an intention-to-treat (ITT) or as per-protocol (PP) approach? Was this appropriate?

Conclusions/Discussion

8.   What were the conclusions drawn?
- o   Are the conclusions valid? (internal validity)
- o   Are the authors trying to make important 'negative' findings seem insignificant? Are they pushing unimportant 'positive' findings to seem significant?
9.   What were the limitations?
- o   Have they clearly addressed the limitations of the study?
- o   Have they possibly misinterpreted correlation for cause?
- o   What work needs to be done moving forward in order to fill in the gaps/add to the literature?
10.   Is the study generalisable to the wider population and clinical practice?
- o   Are the findings and conclusions drawn applicable to the wider population? (external validity)
- o   Are the outcomes strong enough to consider a change to your clinical practice? If not, why?
- o   What are the costs vs benefits? Are the changes economically viable?
11.   What's YOUR conclusion?
- o   What are the strengths/weaknesses of the paper?
- o   What is your overall opinion on the paper?

o   Would you have drawn the same conclusions? Your comments on moving forward?

Once you're familiar with this, memorise the following **condensed framework** of buzzwords to help you recall the questions above:

Title & Introduction/Aims/Objectives/Background

- Study type? Valid research question? Outcomes of interest identified?

Methods

- Suitable sample size and follow-up length? Inclusion/exclusion criteria? Generalisable to population? Sensible control? Randomisation? Confounding variables (and were they accounted for)? Blinded? Ethical considerations?

Results

- Results of interest displayed? Any obviously important results omitted? Confidence levels? Significance? Drop-outs (attrition bias)? ITT vs PP?

Conclusions/Discussion

- Internal validity (valid conclusions)? Limitations (addressed)? Mistaken correlation for cause? External validity (generalisable conclusions)? Likely to change clinical practice? Cost vs benefit analysis? Work needed moving forward?

Critical Appraisal - Time Allocation

As mentioned before, you'll have approximately 15-20 minutes to read your abstract just prior to starting the interview; you'll have to decide how much time you wish to dedicate to each station (e.g. if appraising a study is your weaker topic, you may wish to spend 20 minutes on the abstract and 10 minutes on the clinical scenarios). Albeit the clinical station technically being more important, a lot of candidates may wish to borrow a few minutes of their allotted time to lend it to the abstract appraisal (something most candidates are generally less experienced with). Here is our recommendation on how to allocate your time when receiving the abstract, assuming **15 minutes** are dedicated to this (this is just a suggestion - it goes without saying that preferences will vary a lot between candidates):

Reading the abstract - 2 minutes. This is not to be rushed; do this once and do it properly. With nerves running high in these situations, trying to focus on taking in information will be more difficult than usual. Try to superficially identify the core elements of the study (i.e. intervention group had/did not have a significantly difference outcome of the control etc.) without trying to memorise the details.

Title & Introduction/Aims/Objectives/Background - 2 minute. With practice, this should be an effortless combining of: who authored the study, what the study is briefly about, when and where it was published.

Methods - 4 minutes. Methodology is the keystone of any study; spend time in this section picking up as many flaws in research design, inconsistencies and even important one liners that are placed to seem insignificant.

Results - 2 minutes. This is simply where the results are stated. There may be a few things to pick up in this section, mainly how the results are presented, if they've omitted any outcomes that they've mentioned earlier, loss to follow-up etc.

Conclusions/Discussion - 5 minutes. Just as important as the 'methods' section, you'll need to spend this time evaluating the internal and external validity of the study, the author's concluding remarks and your own thoughts. Use this time to also reflect upon the entire appraisal and how to tie this in to your upcoming presentation.

Presentation Framework

Once we've asked ourselves these questions about the abstract (appraisal), we can then merge these thoughts to present back a slick summary using the following framework:

1. This is a study by *Author et al.* published in *Y Journal* on *publication month/year*.
2. The study is a ***description of study** including study type, ±randomised, ±blinded, ±number of centers, ±trial length, etc.*
3. The **population** of interest was *inclusion criteria*, excluding those who/with *exclusion criteria*
4. The **intervention** group consisted of *describe intervention*.
5. The **control** selected was *describe control*
6. The **outcomes** of interest were *Primary outcome ± secondary outcome ± other outcomes*. The results of the primary outcome were *describe results of intervention group compared with control group*. *Repeat again for other significant outcomes*
7. The things I liked about this abstract were ***strengths** of abstract*. The things I didn't like about it or would like to explore more were ***weaknesses** of abstract ± important omitted information*
8. **Overall**, this abstract *describe the overall impression of the study as per the available abstract. Superficially and quickly touch on unanswered questions regarding methodology, validity of conclusions made from the results displayed and further discussion that needs to be had*

Critical Appraisals & Presentations - Worked Examples

Now, let's use the above frameworks to critically **appraise** some recent RCT abstracts (what you'll be doing on receiving the abstract) and **present** them (the succinct summary you'll mentally prepare for the interviewers):

Please search up the following study abstract online:

ABSTRACT 1: SIX MONTH RANDOMIZED, MULTICENTER TRIAL OF CLOSED-LOOP CONTROL IN TYPE 1 DIABETES - *BROWN ET AL. NEJM. OCTOBER 31, 2019.*

TITLE & BACKGROUND

- Study type: Multicenter RCT.
- Research question: Do closed-loop systems that automate insulin delivery improve glycaemic outcomes in patients with type 1 diabetes compared with sensor-augmented pumps?
- Primary outcome: Percentage of time that the blood glucose level was within the target range of 70 to 180 mg per deciliter (3.9 to 10.0 mmol/liter), as measured by continuous glucose monitoring.
- Secondary outcomes: Percentage of time that the glucose was >180 mg per deciliter, mean glucose levels, glycated haemoglobin, and percentage of time that the glucose level was <70 mg per deciliter or <54 mg per deciliter (3.0 mmol per liter).

METHODS

- Sample size: 168. For a multicenter trial, this is hardly representative of the wider population. What were their baseline characteristics? Were they young, compliant individuals with good diet control? We're unable to establish any confounding variables from this abstract alone, nor can we highlight any selection bias as no recruitment information is available.
- Randomisation: Yes, but no mention of how this was done.
- Follow-up length: 6 months. This is hardly suitable for detection of long-term glycaemic control in a lifelong condition.
- Inclusion/exclusion criteria: N/A apart from having T1DM as inclusion criteria. Age and glycated haemoglobin ranges of the patient sample were mentioned, although I'm unsure if this was consistent with exclusion criteria or simply down to chance of the sample.

- Control group: Use of sensor-augmented pump. Is this the current gold-standard of automated insulin control? If so, this would be a suitable control group.
- Blinding: Not mentioned. We can assume then that at the very least, this study was not double-blinded. Do both intervention and control insulin systems look identical? Unlikely - no mention of a 'double dummy' design so safe to assume this had no participant blinding too. Allocation bias/observer biases introduced? Without blinding, another question is raised: did this RCT omit other expectations from the recommended 'CONSORT' guidelines?

RESULTS

- Primary outcome results were displayed clearly. Select secondary outcomes were also shown. 'No serious hypoglycaemic events occurred in either group' - what is classified as a serious hypoglycaemic event as opposed to a non-serious hypoglycaemic event, does this need elaboration?
- Were there any participant dropouts? - Not mentioned (possible attrition bias if those who withdrew shared certain characteristics, particularly non-compliance). Moreover, was an 'ITT' or 'PP' protocol approach used? Mean values (+- standard deviations) were used. Confidence limits were also included and a strong p value chosen (<0.001).

CONCLUSIONS

- Internal validity: The authors' concluding statement is precise and specific to the trial, supported by the results displayed regarding the primary outcome.
- External validity: No comment made by authors regarding generalisability. As mentioned before, a larger sample size would be needed to represent the wider population (assuming the 168 patients are not completely representative of all type 1 diabetics).
- Limitations (from information available): Only 6-month follow-up (long term outcomes?). Small sample size with a large range of patients (age and glycaemic control).
- Is this slight improvement of glycaemic control worth the adoption of the closed-loop system? Is there a long-term difference in adverse outcomes between the groups? Is the closed-loop system preferred by the users? Is it more difficult to use? Does it cost more, and if so, is it worth it? 'In the closed-loop group, the median percentage of time that the system was in closed-loop

mode was 90% over 6 months.' - Does this mean that the system itself is not entirely accurate? How does this skew results?

- Moving forward, additional large multicenter RCTs need to be carried out to confirm these preliminary findings. Are the results of this trial alone likely to change clinical practice? Unlikely.

Things to note:

1. NEJM trial abstracts tend to be heavy on the methods and results, not so much the background and conclusions. Therefore, the study type, research question, outcomes of interest and conclusions should be fairly straightforward to identify, as these are very clear and precise strips of information. A lot of the 'appraising' will therefore stem from the methods and results; notice there is hardly any mention of discussion (the heading itself is simply 'conclusions'), leaving a lot to be said by you during this stage of the appraisal.
2. Scientific articles do not read like regular journal articles. It is only through repeated engagement in scientific literature that you will start to appreciate common patterns and familiarise yourself with writing styles. If there is one tip you should take away to improve your critical appraisal skill, it would be to read and critique many abstracts in groups and by yourselves.
3. For the appraisal of any RCT, it's good to be aware of the CONSORT guidelines (recommended checklist for RCTs). Ofcourse, CONSORT is expected from the full study and not the abstract, but this is still worth having at the back of your mind.

PRESENTATION

- This study by Brown et al., published in NEJM in October 2019, was a non-blinded, six month randomised multicenter trial of closed-loop control in type-1 diabetes.
- The study was conducted on patients with type 1 diabetes, with no explicit mention of inclusion and exclusion criteria.
- The intervention group saw patients randomised to receive insulin through a closed-loop system. The control group consisted of patients receiving insulin through a sensor-augmented pump.
- The primary outcome of interest was the percentage of time that patients remained between a target range of blood glucose levels, as measured by continuous blood glucose monitoring over the six months. The mean adjusted difference in the intervention group was 11% more time spent in the target blood glucose range after

the 6 months, with a 95% confidence interval of 9-14%, p value of less than 0.001. The control group saw no change over the 6 months, keeping at a 59% time spent within the target range over the 6 months.

- What I liked about this abstract was that it clearly highlights the results of the primary and secondary outcomes, resulting in a succinct conclusion regarding a favourable primary outcome in the intervention group over the control group.
- However, the abstract leaves a lot of questions unanswered, with the overpowering results sections leaving little room for discussion regarding methodology. How were patients recruited? Were any confounding variables adjusted for? Were all patients previously on the sensor-augmented pump, and, if this was unblinded, could any potential treatment difference be simply due to a placebo effect? What are the patient perceptions of this closed-loop system, the cost:benefit analyses?
- These sorts of questions need to be answered in the full paper in order to make further comments on the validity of the conclusions, the study's external validity and considerations moving forwards from this study.

Things to note:

1. Keep the study summary short and sweet, but don't miss out the important core elements (usually covered using an intro to what the paper is about + 'PICO').
2. The NEJM is a popular journal for many AFP critical appraisal stations . This was not an ideal abstract to be given for appraisal, there's not much to comment on besides the studies primary/secondary outcomes and the corresponding results. In this situation, a lot is left to the imagination. Don't feel comfortable if you think the simplicity and clarity of the abstract will work in your favour, the interviewers may just as well spend the entire time talking about what **isn't** in the abstract.
3. Note how the abstract has been summarised succinctly in 4 short points. Anyone can spend endless time breaking down an abstract/study in detail, the difficulty lies in understanding the paper well enough to condense it down to its core elements. Afterwards, the interviewers are sure to explore more concepts in depth, this is where you can pour out the academic details.

ABSTRACT 2: EFFICACY AND SAFETY OF UPADACITINIB IN PATIENTS WITH ACTIVE ANKYLOSING SPONDYLITIS (SELECT-AXIS 1): A MULTICENTRE, RANDOMISED, DOUBLE-BLIND, PLACEBO-CONTROLLED, PHASE 2/3 TRIAL - *VAN DER HEIJDE ET AL, LANCET. NOV 12, 2019.*

TITLE & BACKGROUND

- Study type: A multicentre, randomised, double-blind, placebo-controlled, phase 2/3 trial.
- Outcomes of interest: 'The efficacy and safety of upadacitinib, a selective JAK1 inhibitor, in patients with ankylosing spondylitis.' 'The primary endpoint was the composite outcome measure of the Assessment of SpondyloArthritis international Society 40 response at week 14.'

METHODS
- Sample size: 187 + 178 = 365. Were the patients selected consecutively from hospitals/clinics or otherwise (reduces recruitment bias)? If not, how?
- Inclusion/exclusion criteria: Why were patients who were treated with 'DMARDS' excluded? This is an exclusion of patients with more advanced ankylosing spondylitis, meaning we won't know the true effect of the test drug in this important patient demographic.
- Control: Placebo. Why was a similar medication not used for comparison? If (hypothetically), upadacitinib had a positive treatment effect compared to the placebo of two-fold, should this hold merit if the current alternatives have a four-fold effect? Just because it's better than the placebo, doesn't necessarily make it a good treatment!
- Blinding: Double-blind.
- Randomisation: 'Patients were randomly assigned 1:1 using interactive response technology.' (Don't worry, we have no idea what this means either).

FINDINGS
- Intention to treat protocol used - 'Analyses were done in the full analysis set of patients who were randomly assigned and received at least one dose of study drug.' Therefore, no attrition bias.
- Results showed confidence intervals and a significant p-value. However, the treatment difference between intervention and control groups can be as small as 13% as per the 95% CI. If you

were a patient, would this influence your choice to take the new medication over no medication?

- 'One serious adverse event was reported in each group'. Excluding the placebo group, what was the serious adverse event in the intervention group? Was it a known side effect? What is the risk of that event occurring with the drug? Does it demerit the positive findings of the study?
- Regarding the common adverse effect of raised creatine phosphokinase, to what extent was this raised? How would patients be advised to counter this effect? What are the ethical considerations if these were known significant side effects?

INTERPRETATION

- Internal validity: Upadacitinib was 'efficacious' - acceptable conclusion (albeit only compared with placebo). Upadacitinib was 'well tolerated' - 62% of patients experienced adverse events, this needs to be explored more before validating this conclusion. Were these 'adverse events' relatively innocent? This study supports 'the further investigation of upadacitinib for the treatment of axial spondyloarthritis'? Arguably not. Firstly, it must be clarified that this treatment is suitable only in the case of intolerance, contraindication or poor response to anti-inflammatory drugs (as per what was tested). Additionally, if the current recommended guidelines are to escalate these patients onto DMARDs (which may have stronger treatment effect and/or less adverse events), why should upadacitinib be considered further?
- External validity: The study was double blinded and recruited a large cohort from multiple centres and different countries, this is likely to be generalisable to the wider population.
- Limitations (from information available): Not tested in patients using DMARDs. Placebo used as control as compared to current guideline-recommended drug. Confounding variables - were the patients on other medications? Were these accounted for?
- Cost vs benefit analysis: N/A. Would this study (abstract) make me consider a change to my clinical practice? Unlikely. There is simply not enough information available regarding its efficacy and side effects compared to the current recommended treatment. Also, what are the patient perceptions of the drug, would they consider the treatment difference worthy of the downsides of the medication? More robust studies need to be carried before concluding that upadacitinib warrants further investigation for its use in ankylosing spondylitis.

Things to note:
1. There's no way you'd be able to appraise all of this within the time frame, we know. These breakdowns are to highlight the potential points you may wish to address and how you could potentially address them. As the interviewers are unlikely to dwell on the appraisal for too long, you will either have time to address **your** points of interest (stronger position for you - dig deep into the critical points you've considered), or, they'll directly question on you on **their** points of interest (through prior practice, pattern recognition will allow you recite similar, suitable answers).
2. On receiving the abstract, make sure to highlight and annotate as much as possible. Then, we recommend writing the appraisal headings on the side, using short keywords to remind yourself of all the different talking points for quick reference in the interview. E.g. 'recruitment bias?'; 'control = placebo?'; 'DMARD users not included?', etc.
3. Compared with the previous NEJM abstract, you may agree that there are more holes to point out in the methodology/conclusions drawn in this abstract. In these situations, it's easy to doubt oneself over whether you've actually identified flaws in such a high-impact factor journal study, questioning one's own academic authority. The truth is that there are always flaws. Say what you think and more importantly, say it with confidence. Do not hesitate when 'ripping apart' a paper, it shows a strong understanding of methodology, critical thinking and logical deduction. And, the more you cover, the less the interviewers need to ask.

PRESENTATION
- This is a multicentre, randomised, double-blind, placebo-controlled, phase 2/3 trial by Van der Heijde et al. looking at the efficacy and safety of upadacitinib in patients with active ankylosing spondylitis.
- The **population** of interest was patients with ankylosing spondylitis who had an inadequate response to or unable to take NSAIDS. Patients excluded from the study included: those previously treated with DMARDS and those who did not fulfill the modified New York criteria.
- The **intervention** group took 15mg of oral upadacitinib once daily for a 14-week period, whilst the **control** group took an oral placebo tablet/capsule.
- The first **outcome** of interest was the primary endpoint of the composite measure of the Assessment of SpondyloArthritis international Society 40 response at week 14. The intervention

group had the aforementioned response 26% more than that of the control group, with 95% confidence intervals noted and a significant p-value.

- Another **outcome** of interest was upadacitinib's safety, measured by the frequency and severity of adverse incidents in the intervention group. The abstract mentions a slight increase in adverse events in the intervention group (62% of patients) compared with the control group (55% of patients).
- Notably, before I can think of any immediate strengths of this abstract, there are some important questions left to be answered: Why were patients treated with DMARDs excluded from the study? Does this correlate with an exclusion of patients with more severe ankylosing spondylitis? Why was a placebo used for the control group as opposed to the current recommended drug for these patients?
- Moreover, the internal validity of the conclusions drawn can be questioned here, particularly that of upadacitinib being an efficacious drug and warranting further investigation for its use in the treatment of ankylosing spondylitis. A deeper dive into the full study is needed to further evaluate the study design's core methodological decisions, before further discussion can be had regarding the papers external validity and conclusions.

Things to note:
1. The introduction to presenting the abstract is usually just a rearrangement of the title, authors, journal and first section of the abstract (aims/introduction/background etc.).
2. The second to last bullet point (above) **superficially** touches on some points that we've considered beforehand, inviting the interviewer to now explore those comments further through questioning. This is a technique known as 'leading the interview', finishing your answers in a way that can be seamlessly followed up by questions from the interviewer. Contrast this with an abrupt ending to the presentation (without the final bullet point), the interviewer can now ask almost any question he/she likes, potentially throwing you off guard. By setting up for the interviewer to follow up on your points, you remain in control of the topics and can really nail the answers (after all, you mentioned them because you've already thought about them!).

How To Practice This Section

It goes without saying that you should be practicing your interview stations as much as (if not more than) hitting the books. Many of you will not have been formally interviewed since your application to medical school. This sets the default standard very low and therefore, allows interviewers to witness a broad spectrum of interview prowess between those who don't prepare and those aiming to set the bar high. The problem is, almost every applicant will take the interview preparation seriously, it's up to you to ensure that your preparation is more robust and timely than that of the competition.

Generally, it wouldn't make sense to recommend preparing for an interview you haven't yet been offered. However, AFP interviews can often be thrown upon you at very short notice, so it's best to get familiar with the following sections and really 'step on the gas' if and when you receive an invitation to interview.

There are several different facets to preparing for this station effectively. First of all, you need to familiarise yourself with key terms and concepts. Read our academic glossary and practice explaining concepts to non-medical friends and family. As the saying goes, "If you can't explain it to a 6-year old, you don't know it yourself." Instead of simply reciting a definition verbatim, try and explain the term in the context of its use in a paper that you've recently read.

Reading a research paper is fairly straightforward; critically appraising a paper requires an active mental effort to pick holes in it using common sense and an understanding of research methodology. Luckily, the AFP academic station only requires the appraisal of a research paper's abstract. Practising with your peers for this station can be formal or informal, as long as you're scrutinising each other's answers and really digging out their understanding, so consider picking up the latest issue of a popular journal (NEJM, Lancet etc.) and see how much you can talk about/appraise the paper by simply reading the abstract.

Here's a great tip if you know someone 'medical' who's willing to practice with you: Each of you study a paper and then exchange abstracts (to be appraised after 10-20 minutes of reading). In this way, you'll be blind to the new abstract (mimicking the real scenario) and an expert examiner for your peer (mimicking the position of the interview panel). You could even replicate this in a group setting over coffee, garnering constructive criticism from multiple sources in a single sitting.

As mentioned before, make sure to question each other about what specific terms mean (double-blind, confidence interval etc.) and their practical application in the context of the study. Remember, you'll have no more than 30 minutes to read your abstract and clinical scenario before your interview stations begin, so have a think about how much time you want to allocate to the abstract. We would recommend erring on the side of caution during practice, so try and give yourself a few minutes less to account for all the nerves on the big day.

Chapter 5 - Interview Practice

5.1 - Personal Questions

1. Tell me about yourself.
2. Take me through your CV.
3. Describe your clinical experience to date.
4. Describe your research experience to date.
5. Tell me about your most significant research project.
6. Why do you enjoy research?
7. What are the qualities of a good researcher?
8. Describe your teaching experience to date.
9. Tell me about your most memorable teaching experience.
10. Why do you enjoy teaching?
11. What are the qualities of a good teacher?
12. Tell me about your experience of working within a team.
13. Tell me about your experience in leading a team.
14. What is your main strength?
15. What is your main weakness?
16. What is your proudest achievement?
17. How do you cope with stress?
18. Where do you see yourself in 5-10 years?
19. Talk me through your clinical and academic aspirations.

5.2 - Clinical Station

1. You are an F1 on a night shift covering 9 wards. You attend a patient who has received an infusion of antibiotics containing penicillin, despite being allergic to penicillin. He has become tachypnoeic and his blood pressure has dropped from 115/80 to 100/65. It is just you and two nurses available on the ward. (a) What would you do next? (b) What would be your management plan?

2. You are an F1 on a night shift covering 9 wards. You are suddenly bleeped 3 times. The first bleep is from a nurse who wishes for you to sign the prescription of a patient's antibiotics that was due 30 minutes ago. The second bleep is from a nurse that has just reported a suspected and unwitnessed fall (65 year old man with dementia found on the floor a few metres from his bed). The third bleep is regarding a patient who has a NEWS score of 5, the nurse is new to the ward and

is concerned about her. Who would you attend first and what is your reasoning?

3. You are an F1 who is due to clerk a patient admitted into the acute medical unit. Your patient, David Smith, is a 55 year old man who has come in with acute shortness of breath. He has recently come back from a roadtrip across the UK, claiming he has also coughed up some phlegm over the last couple of hours, although he did not note the colour and claims this can be normal for him. His past medical history consists of: hypertension, hypercholesterolaemia, rheumatoid arthritis, COPD and anaemia. He is allergic to co-amoxiclav. He has a strong history of smoking, lives at home with his wife and two pets. (a) What are your next steps and management plan? (b) What are your top differentials?

4. You are an F1 who has just received a bleep review a patient with a K+ of 6.6. Upon arrival, you see dynamic changes on a recently performed ECG. (a) What changes are you likely to see on the ECG? (b) What would be your next steps and management plan?

5. You are an F1 who has just reviewed an abdominal X-ray for a patient with severe abdominal pain and distension. You think you see grossly dilated bowel loops in the film. It's 6pm and most ward doctors have gone home. (a) What are your next steps and your management plan?

5.3 - Academic Station

1. Why do you want to do the AFP?
2. Why do you want to do the AFP here?
3. Why do you want to do an AFP on this topic?
4. What makes you the right AFP candidate?
5. What challenges do you anticipate from the programme? How do you plan on overcoming them?
6. What will you do if are not successful in attaining a place on the programme?
7. What you know about the integrated academic training pathway?
8. How do you think a clinical academic career differs to that of a normal clinician?
9. What do you hope to accomplish through your research?
10. What are your academic (research) aspirations?
11. What do you understand by the pyramid of evidence in research?
12. What is a p-value?

13. What is a confidence interval?
14. What is the power of a study and why is it important?
15. What is a Kaplan-Meier curve?
16. What is a forest plot?
17. What is the purpose of blinding in a study?
18. What is bias and why is it relevant to research?
19. What is intention-to-treat analysis?
20. What is the 'number needed to treat' and why is it useful?
21. What is the difference between sensitivity and specificity?
22. Tell me about a paper you've recently read including its strengths and weaknesses
23. What sort of critical questions must one ask when reading a study?
24. Why do studies need to be peer-reviewed?
25. What are the most important components of a study?
26. How does research lead to changes in clinical practice?
27. Do you think all published research is good research?
28. What is the difference between research and quality improvement?
29. What is the difference between audit and quality improvement?
30. What is an audit?
31. Do you think all doctors should be required to participate in research?
32. Do you think all healthcare staff should be required to participate in audit or quality improvement?
33. Why do you think it is important for a study protocol to be published before the study?

Chapter 6 - Advice from AFP Doctors

To make this handbook as representative as possible, we reached out to AFP doctors from across the UK to answer a set of questions. The questions and answers will either: provide advice on how to prepare for the AFP as an 'early stage' medical student, help you decide which AUoA to apply for, highlight what is expected from each AUoA, provide unique advice on how each successful applicant prepared or, provide talking points for your interviews.

Here are the 7 questions we asked:

1. **What unique factors about your AUoA do you think prospective applicants would benefit from knowing about in advance?**
2. **Can you please provide a brief overview of your experience at the interview in your AUoA(s)?**
3. **What were, in your opinion, the best things you did that helped you attain an AFP post? Is there anything you would have done differently looking back?**
4. **Since applying for your AFP post, have you learnt anything new about the post worth sharing, either positive or negative?**
5. **What are the most important pieces of advice you would share with an applicant currently applying to the AFP?**
6. **What advice would you give to medical students who still have a long time to prepare for the AFP?**
7. **What were your top resources when applying for the AFP?**

Below, you will find a compilation of answers kindly provided by current or former AFP doctors, with their respective names and positions:

1. **What unique factors about your AUoA do you think prospective applicants would benefit from knowing about in advance?**

"My [research block in FY2] was not an entirely academic block as it required us to act as the cardiothoracic SHO 1 in 2 weekends. The programme allowed for numerous teaching and research collaboration opportunities."

- Dr Azeem Alam - Surgery AFP at St Thomas' Hospital

"I have been offered a full scholarship for a £3000 PgCert. My academic supervisor allowed me to tailor my research interests, which is not immediately apparent when applying for the London AFP. I would advise any prospective applicants to email their supervisor if they believe they like the programme but feel reluctant to do the research that is advertised. It may be that you don't get a reply but it's well worth a shot if it means you get to pick an AFP that combines your favourite clinical rotations with your preferred academic interests. St George's also offer the opportunity for anyone to become involved in regular teaching of clinical skills, anatomy, etc. This can be a valuable experience both for your CV and professional development."

- Dr Miguel Sequeira Campos - Plastic Surgery AFP at St George's Hospital

"The programme is very flexible and trailed to trainee's interests. It offers the opportunity to work with NICE in London. You can choose an integrated academic block as part of a leadership AFP, or 4 month block as part of a research AFP."

- Dr Vageesh Jain - Public Health AFP in Leicester

"This Academic Block allows you to get involved in teaching medical students across a range of primary care and population health areas (E.g. dermatology, women's health, etc). UCL offers free training in teaching and support to gain higher teaching accreditation if so inclined. There is a dedicated 4 month research block based at the Royal Free Hospital, whilst FY2 clinical rotations are based at Whittington."

- Dr Shyam Gokani - Primary Care and Population Health AFP at UCL

"Yorkshire & Humber offers 66 AFP places across three regions, which operate autonomously, enabling applicants to tailor their interview preparation to the city they desire. Within Y&H there are 48 research AFPs in addition to 3-primary care specific AFPs in West Yorkshire. These research posts are not specialty-specific, which provides the benefit of enabling trainees to self-design a project in their area of research interest or to select a project from a predesigned list. Notably, Y&H has one of the largest and most established Medical Education AFP programmes within the UK, with three medical education posts based at the University of Hull and 12 posts based at the University of Sheffield. All trainees entering the research AFP will be enrolled on a fully funded postgraduate certificate in Health Research, whilst trainees in entering the medical education AFP will be enrolled on a fully funded postgraduate certificate in Health Professionals Education (in East Yorkshire) or Medical Education (in South Yorkshire)."

"Specific insider info to Sheffield Medical Education AFP:

It has been running for many years and, in 2019, the content of the postgraduate Certificate in Medical Education was completely revamped to account for the latest innovations in medical education. The PgCert itself is very manageable and requires two full days of training with two essays over three four-month rotations. Two of these blocks will be during FY1 and the third will be during your allocated teaching block in FY2. Additionally, in your FY2 year, you are given the freedom to either design a teaching course/programme for a student selected component at Sheffield Medical School or undertake a research project related to medical education. This flexibility is great as it accommodates for individual with a particular interest in curriculum development and also individuals who would like to gain more research experience whilst getting experience in medical education for their CV. The Four month teaching block in FY2 has three main types of teaching - anatomy demonstration, clinical teaching and pre-clinical tutorials. The specific topics within these teaching types will vary depending on the time of year your academic slot is location. For example, if your teaching slot is in the second rotation of FY2 you will be teaching neuroanatomy in the anatomy block and if your teaching slot is in the third rotation you will be teaching finals OSCEs preparation in the clinical slot."

"Specific Pros of the Sheffield Medical Education AFP:
Opportunity to demonstrate anatomy; fully-funded PgCert in Medication Education; Large cohort of Medical Education AFP trainees (12), who study alongside other doctors on the PgCert, which allows you to form a close group of friends group; Opportunity to undertake either curriculum design or a medical education research project; Based at a University with a strong research environment; Based in a young city with a great mix of cheap restaurants, bars and countryside activities."

- Dr Ciaran Kennedy - Medical Education AFP at the University of Sheffield

"There were a number of factors that made West Yorkshire's Academic Foundation Programme stand out.
Firstly, I wanted the option to seek out/design my own AFP project, rather than choose one from a pre-selected list and in West Yorkshire we had the freedom to do this. This is particularly useful if you know what you would like to focus on for your four-month research block, or if you already have some contacts in the area that you would like to start/continue working with.

Additionally, the West Yorkshire academic foundation posts offer free enrolment in the Postgraduate Certificate in Health Research at the University of Leeds. This is an additional qualification that provides teaching time to develop valuable research skills.
Finally, it's not just about the AFP. Think about the city you'll be living and working in for the next two years. Leeds is a great city, with excellent teaching hospitals. Great football team too."

- Dr Joseph P Thompson - Neurosurgery AFP at Leeds Hospitals Trust

"The FY2 Academic year is made up of two 6 month clinical placements. One in gastroenterology, and the other in a specialty of your choice. The academic time (total equivalent to one 4 month block), is spread throughout the year. You also undertake a Postgraduate Certificate in 'Healthcare Leadership Management and Innovation' and have ample time to work on Projects."

- Dr Rebecca Lissmann - Leadership and Management AFP in South West

"Two unique factors are: (1) Intensive care rotation. One of the least demanding from a timing perspective with 40 hours a week of work on a fixed predetermined schedule. This is an excellent opportunity to take time to study for any additional qualifications that may be coming up (I personally used this to study for the MRCS). In addition, the rotation offers a protected learning environment for developing skills that you would not have the opportunity to practice on any other rotations (Eg. central and arterial lines). There are always seniors around as well, which is particularly helpful as you are handling the sickest patients in the hospital. (2) Plastic surgery rotation. This may change but this was the only AFP in London which offered a Plastic Surgery rotation. In addition, meeting with previous junior doctors who have had this job, it sounds like > 90% of your time is spent in theatres, and you often get to perform minor procedures in their entirety. Great team as well."

- Dr Xi Ming Zhu - General Practice AFP at St. George's Hospital

"Fully funded place for the Post Graduate Certificate in health research at the University of Leeds, and the opportunity to decide exactly what speciality you do your project in."

- Dr Harry Hodgson - Trauma & Orthopaedic Surgery AFP in Yorkshire & Humber

"(1) Sponsored Postgraduate Certificate in Health Research and Statistics at the University of York, to be carried out part-time over 2 years. It will be a PGCert in Medical Education instead if you're doing an 'education' academic placement. (2) Dedicated 4-month research block with 1 in 6 weekends covering the ambulatory care unit (ample time to get Horus eportfolio up to scratch and it bumps your pay up slightly). (3) Opportunities to help out with mock AFP interviews for final year medical students."

- Dr Efioanwan Andah - Primary Care AFP in Yorkshire and Humber

"(1) Opportunity to be a clinical skills tutor and anatomy demonstrator (2) PGCert with funding available"

- Dr Eyal Ben-David - Renal AFP at St George's Hospital

"Working in a tertiary centre that is situated beside a medical school. The medical school are always looking for junior doctors to assist with teaching and examining. Opportunities include: being an anatomy demonstrator, clinical skills tutor, medical school interviewer and OSCE examiner. Those with a keen interest in teaching can further their interest by completing formal qualifications such as a PGCert during their foundation years at St. George's. There are other opportunities to build your teaching portfolio through bedside teaching, revision lectures for medical schools and assisting in conferences held by the various societies at St. George's, University of London. St. George's has plenty of exciting research which committed academic junior doctors can get involved in. This does require the junior doctor to be proactive and actively reach out to the researchers / consultants / professors of the specialty's department."

- Dr Saeed Azizi - General Practice AFP at St George's Hospital

2. Can you please provide a brief overview of your experience at the interview in your AUoA(s)?

"The interview was 1 hour long. You are given an abstract to critically appraise and a clinical scenario. The first 30 minutes allowed for 15 minutes to prepare the critical appraisal and the second 15 minutes to read through the scenario. I would encourage you to take as many notes as possible during this time as you can be thrown off track once in front of the examiners. Split your time equally and ensure you have a structured and logical approach to critical appraisal. My abstract was discussing various new peri-operative antiseptic agents. Assessing the clinical scenario requires you to think about differential diagnoses, investigation options (bedside, bloods, imaging, invasive tests), and management options. Be sure to also brush up on your pathophysiology as my scenario was DKA and I was asked numerous questions on this and its pathophysiological difference to HHS. Learn the key medical and surgical emergencies inside out."

- Dr Azeem Alam - Surgery AFP at St Thomas' Hospital

"LONDON: From what I recall, my interview was in the second available slot in the morning. It also took place during the earliest possible date of the 3 that London made available. I wore a suit and tie and made sure to sleep well the night before. I don't think I had much appetite so ended up doing the interview on an empty stomach so, looking back, it would have been nice to have made myself eat something. I arrived nice and early and walked into a room that had 2 people checking IDs at the front and was already full of applicants who were waiting. I signed in and had to wait around for quite a while. I spoke to some of the other applicants (although many chose to sit in silence). Eventually I had my ID checked and waited a while longer to be called in as they were running late. When I was called in, we walked in a small group to another room where we sat in exam conditions.

There was a timer on a projector and we were all given 25 minutes to appraise a clinical abstract (with 3 scenarios) and an academic abstract. I had another sheet of A4 but chose to make my annotations directly on the paper that had the abstracts. When the time was up we were called out of the room and onto the corridor where we sat in front of our corresponding doors before going in - pretty similar to an OSCE. My first station was the clinical, where I had 2 examiners. I went through what I had planned during the waiting period and explained my thought process. They seemed pleased with what I was saying and barely asked me anything extra. My second station was the academic one, again with 2 examiners. I had a personal question about my academic interests and then was asked to appraise the abstract. I mainly followed the questions they asked as they were very specific and they didn't seem to want me run through my own framework for abstract appraisal. There were no complicated questions about statistics and most of the questions seemed to delve into whether I understood the meaning of the abstract and could contextualise it's significance to the field. I left the interview feeling pleased, if uncertain as to how exactly I had done.

WALES: I had my university Immediate Life Support session the day before my interview, which was a bit inconvenient. After it was done, I hopped on a train down to Wales. I spent the night at a hotel and left early in the morning for my interview. When I arrived at the venue, I was greeted and directed to a waiting room. I met a few other applicants and we waited together until we were called in. I waited outside the first door until I was called in to what was my clinical station. I had 3 examiners and they gave me 2 clinical scenarios. I was supposed to have split my time in half but the examiners apparently forgot to start the timer (which they apologised for at the end) and I ended up spending about 7-8 minutes in the first scenario (as they kept asking increasingly detailed questions) and just 1-2 minutes for the second. Once I realised what had happened, I had to make it clear that I would be safe under time pressure. This meant that for the 2nd scenario, rather than beginning with a standard A-E, I used the clinical history I was provided and informed them of the most urgent differential diagnoses I would look to rule out in the immediate setting. I then told them what steps (including investigations) I would take and suggested the most likely diagnoses based on the few values they had the time to provide me with. I believe that, despite the lack of time, I presented a sensible range of differential diagnoses and managed to showcase my clinical acumen. I think they appreciated the fact that I was able to think on my feet and not get flustered by the issue with timings. My second station was the academic station. Again, I had 3 examiners and each of them asked 1 question. The questions were pretty straight forward and I made an effort to present myself as calm and composed, with a logical and structured thought process to each of my answers. My main reason for applying for the Wales AFP was the fact they have the largest Plastic Surgery research center in the UK and I made sure to put across this motivation in my answers, which I am certain weighed in my favour when they decided. It was all over pretty quickly and I was satisfied with my performance even though it was difficult to say exactly how well I'd done."

- Dr Miguel Sequeira Campos - Plastic Surgery AFP at St George's Hospital

"30 minute interview with 2 stations - (1) Research ethics and designing a study/who would you want on a research team, etc. Then some questions on teamwork/leadership. (2) Presenting a paper (which they send before the interview) and answering questions afterwards mostly on methodology/limitations and application."

- Dr Vageesh Jain - Public Health AFP in Leicester

"The London AFP interview consisted of a clinical scenario provided beforehand, with follow up questions. The academic interview was based around discussion of a pre-allocated journal article and your academic motivations."

- Dr Shyam Gokani - Primary Care and Population Health AFP at UCL

"The day consisted of two stations - one academic and one clinical. Each station was around 10 minutes in length with a 5 minute break before the academic station and a 5 minute reading time before the clinical station. The academic station involved asking questions related to your interest in research or medical education, your prior experience in these fields, your ability to cope with the demands of the AFP and instances where you have demonstrated important transferable skills such as teamwork and leadership. The clinical station involved a standard A to E scenario where you were asked to talk through your acute management, act on any investigation findings you were provided (after requesting them), providing a list of different diagnoses, then discussing your management plan and when you would escalate.

There were no attempts to trip you up in either station, nor was there an interviewer acting as 'bad cop'. I felt that this was a more amicable style of interviewing than I have previously experienced and I think that it was more conducive to expressing your achievements and made you feel that you could work with these colleagues in the future."

- Dr Ciaran Kennedy - Medical Education AFP at the University of Sheffield

"There were three stations.

One: I was asked in advance to prepare a brief presentation on 'My interest in Management and Leadership', followed by a typical job interview questioning, which featured broader questions on key issues in healthcare leadership.

Two: Critical discussion of a paper

Three: Clinical scenario"

- Dr Rebecca Lissmann - Leadership and Management AFP in South West

"Large RCT comparing standard 5-year SERM versus new 10-year SERM for treatment of breast cancer. Clinical station is an expected triaging, investigations, and treatment of 4 patients.

Clinical (I got 10/10) - Always focus on who the sickest person is. There are many issues that need to be attended to eventually but do NOT require immediate attention. Read through the entire emergency section of the Oxford Handbook and remember the treatments. My examiners, though friendly, did not offer a single question or advice and I had to fill the entire 10 minutes without prompt. They were smiling for mine, but have heard more stern, blank faces for others who have done very well as well so do not let their reactions guide your confidence about performance on the station.

Academic (I got 9/10) - So the abstract I got had loads of numbers and data. Honestly one of the longest abstracts I've read. Don't get flustered. Much like A to E for assessing an acutely unwell patient, refer to your system, whatever it may be. Talk about what you've read, provide a purpose for the study, the summary of outcomes, and your impression of it. Analyze it using whatever system works for you, some people like going through PICOs, but there are plenty of easy to find systems if you just google it. Use a system of critique and analysis that you like. Also don't make jokes like I did during the station."

- Dr Xi Ming Zhu - General Practice AFP at St. George's Hospital

"Two stations lasting ~10 minutes, one clinical requiring talking through the assessment and management of a common emergency, and an academic station with standard interview questions. Nothing unusual or unexpected!"

- Dr Harry Hodgson - Trauma & Orthopaedic Surgery AFP in Yorkshire & Humber

"The interview consisted of 2 stations which were 15 mins each. The first one was a research/academic station with some data interpretation from a paper and questions about my research interests, my reasons for applying for an AFP, disadvantages and advantages of doing an AFP etc. The other was a clinical station about an elderly gentleman who had a fall on the ward (PS: don't forget your ABCDE approach and to check if they're on any anticoagulation therapy in this particular case!)"

- Dr Efioanwan Andah - Primary Care AFP in Yorkshire and Humber

"The interview consisted of two 10-minute stations (academic and clinical). You are given an abstract and a clinical scenario and a total of 30-minutes to prepare. You can choose how to utilise those 30-minutes. Personally, I dedicated 20-minutes to the abstract and 10-minutes to the clinical scenario. From what I have heard, there is some variation in the style of the interview. I will describe my experience.

My first station was the academic one. There were two interviewers who started by asking me a few personal questions about my reasons for applying to the AFP and about my research experience. I then had to describe the abstract and discuss its strengths and weaknesses. In this station I was basically talking the whole time. The interviewers asked me some simple, open-ended questions but for the most part, I was given free-reign to take the interview to where I wanted it to go. My advice for this station would be to familiarise yourself with study designs and basic statistics. It is important to become comfortable reading medical research and the only way to do this is by practicing.

The clinical station was very different. I was immediately asked to discuss my approach to the clinical scenario. I was interrupted many times and asked quite difficult questions. It's extremely important to know how to do a thorough primary assessment of an unwell patient. It is also important to contextualise this to the clinical scenario. Everyone will have a spiel for their A-E assessment but in order to stand out you need to make it specific to the patient they are asking about. I was asked to discuss and rationalise my differential diagnoses. The key to this is a very logical and structured approach. It is much more impressive if you can categorise your differentials in an intelligent way than if you can just list 10 unrelated differentials in no particular order. The most important thing for this station is a solid foundation of knowledge, clarity of thought and understanding your limitations. If you are unsafe, you will fail, so it is much better to seek senior support than to guess and take risks (this is also important in real life!)."

- Dr Eyal Ben-David - Renal AFP at St George's Hospital

"My understanding is that all applicants to AFPs in London have a similar interview and there is no distinction made on the particular AFP you have applied. I.e those who apply for an AFP in GP will have a similar interview to those who apply for an AFP in medical education.

My experience with the London AFP interview was overall positive. You are invited to attend the interview location at a particular date / time and will have a briefing on the day of the structure of the interview. Like other AFP interviews, the interview consists of two stations, a clinical and academic station. Prior to the stations you are given 30 minutes to read through the clinical scenario and abstract that you will be appraising.

The clinical scenario typically will involve some form of clinical emergency scenario and the research station will typically involve an abstract you will be expected to critically appraise. Interviewers will actively ask questions or may request clarifications for answers. The stations are 10 minutes each and the interview can feel somewhat fast-paced."

- Dr Saeed Azizi - General Practice AFP at St George's Hospital

3.   What were, in your opinion, the best things you did that helped you attain an AFP post? Is there anything you would have done differently looking back?

105

"Mock AFP interviews at KCL. Having friends who have gone through the process already to read and appraise my white space questions, offer advice and recommend books."

- Dr Azeem Alam - Surgery AFP at St Thomas' Hospital

"Plan my time well as there were many demands. Start preparing well in advance. Surrounding myself with the right people who encouraged me to work hard."

- Dr Miguel Sequeira Campos - Plastic Surgery AFP at St George's Hospital

"Managing to obtain publications and presentations; having extra-curricular achievements to talk about during the interview. If I could do it again, I would have read more about research ethics/ the research process to do better in the interview."

- Dr Vageesh Jain - Public Health AFP in Leicester

"It is important to practice with friends and attend all your medical school placements and teaching to gain valuable clinical experience that will help you in your interview. Training to be a good FY1 is part and parcel of the interview preparation and some of this can only be gained from the wards. Finals revision can also be helpful in some cases. If I could do it again, I would probably focus less on knowledge acquisition and more on practice and clinical experience."

- Dr Shyam Gokani - Primary Care and Population Health AFP at UCL

"1) I googled past AFP questions and wrote model answers to learn. Common areas involved your interest in academic medicine, your transferable skills and your ability to cope with stress/a high workload.
2) I learned and practiced aloud the common emergency A->E managements.
3) I revised some basics of stats and research such as 'what are P-Values' and 'the hierarchy of evidence'. It was also worth looking at the pros and cons of various study designs (e.g. Case-Control and Cohort) and ensuring you know the difference between these types."

- Dr Ciaran Kennedy - Medical Education AFP at the University of Sheffield

"Presentations, prizes and publications are all very valuable. When there are compulsory research modules or projects at university make sure that you put in a bit more work to try to get the maximum output from the opportunity. When selecting projects ask your potential supervisor to be realistic about the prospect of publication and timescale etc.
Depending on where you apply, teaching and leadership experience may also be very useful. There are normally many opportunities for teaching whilst at medical school- make sure you embrace these, collect certificates, and try to organise teaching yourself as this can also demonstrate leadership."

- Dr Joseph P Thompson - Neurosurgery AFP at Leeds Hospitals Trust

"A) In terms of experience, I applied for lots of things - and was successful with some. I developed a habit of saying 'yes' to opportunities. This snowballed throughout the course of medical school.
Whilst preparing for the interview, I developed a clear understanding of why I wanted the job, and where I want to go in my career. I had the chance to talk to communicate that passion during the presentation section.
I spoke to contacts who had academic jobs within medicine, and asked them for support throughout the process.
B) I would have prepared more for the 'critical discussion of a paper' section. I had an incorrect perception that it was less important because this was not an academic research post."

- Dr Rebecca Lissmann - Leadership and Management AFP in South West

"I think much of why I got the position I wanted is due to prior work. Having a master's degree, along with previous publications, conference oral and poster presentations absolutely buffered my points. That being said, you can't rest on your laurels. The interviews are still the highest weighted section (140 of 283 possible points), and you need to prepare because that will literally make the biggest difference. Practice, practice, practice with friends."
- Dr Xi Ming Zhu - General Practice AFP at St. George's Hospital

"Revised management of common emergencies and practiced talking through assessment of management of these with friends"
- Dr Harry Hodgson - Trauma & Orthopaedic Surgery AFP in Yorkshire & Humber

"I spoke to current AFP doctors at the time for advice on applications and interviews
I attended a mock interview and AFP prep events, some of which I organised myself as part of the research/academia interest society at my medical school
At this point, I wouldn't have done anything differently looking back."
- Dr Efioanwan Andah - Primary Care AFP in Yorkshire and Humber

"As I didn't have a Bsc, I needed to score a lot of points in other areas. The best thing I did was present all of my work at conferences. Any academic work you do at medical school, including your selected study modules should be submitted to a conference."
- Dr Eyal Ben-David - Renal AFP at St George's Hospital

"The things I did in my preparation which I felt had the highest yield from first to last are listed below.
For the clinical station:
-        Mock interviews with current AFPs where I would practice talking through the presentations, investigations and detailed management of clinical emergencies.
-        Practicing your ABCDE for emergencies in detail and knowing how to fluently talk through this.
-        Oxford Handbook of Clinical Medicine, the final chapter on clinical emergencies is excellent.
For the academic station:
-        Mock interviews with current AFPs where I would be given an abstract to read through and appraise, receiving feedback on areas of improvement.
-        Reading an abstract a day and practicing critically appraising this under timed conditions at home
-        There are plenty of resources online regarding critically appraising papers. What I personally found most helpful were critical appraisal toolkits / checklists."
- Dr Saeed Azizi - General Practice AFP at St George's Hospital

4.   Since applying for your AFP post, have you learnt anything new about the post worth sharing, either positive or negative?

"Positives - The AFP I applied for was in Surgery, and this was later narrowed down to Vascular Surgery. It has allowed me to present at national and international conferences, obtain research and travel grants independently, publish novel research in several peer-reviewed journals, and collaborate across numerous sites such as Public Health England (PHE). The project was largely outlined by my supervisor already so there wasn't much room to change the topic. In my opinion, this allowed for greater focus and to delve into an extremely interesting area of vascular surgery that I had never explored before. The project was largely independent and involved a lot of travel between London and PHE in Oxford, as well as a significant amount of theatre time. I learned a whole new area of medical physics and radiation exposure, which never would have been possible without a dedicated research post. Great colleagues and department!

Negatives - 1 in 4 full weekends covering Cardiothoracics at Guy's Hospital. In reality, these were actually quite enjoyable!."

- Dr Azeem Alam - Surgery AFP at St Thomas' Hospital

"The projects are flexible and you can look for opportunities outside of your department within UCL. To get the most out of your block you need to start preparing well in advance, but not too early. (Ideally 6 months before, depending on the type of project). It really helps to know what specialty you want to go into so try to decide this early with taster weeks, etc. in FY1 or medical school. "

- Dr Shyam Gokani - Primary Care and Population Health AFP at UCL

"The Medical Education AFP is less time-consuming than I first thought and has been designed well to fit around your rota, which is reassuring."

- Dr Ciaran Kennedy - Medical Education AFP at the University of Sheffield

"It may not be something to worry about during foundation years, but if you know what you want to specialise in (and wish to pursue the academic pathway after AFP) then it may be beneficial to apply to an AUoA which has a well-established research group in your chosen field."

- Dr Joseph P Thompson - Neurosurgery AFP at Leeds Hospitals Trust

"There is total free range in terms of project choice.

The four Academic Leadership F1 and F2s have breakfast meetings roughly fortnightly with one of the Medical Directors. This has been an invaluable mentoring space.

In recent years, the Academic Leadership F2s have planned and chaired the South West Trainees Leadership Conference."

- Dr Rebecca Lissmann - Leadership and Management AFP in South West

"So the biggest perk of my AFP, and I think this is often overlooked, is the location. Tooting Broadway is a pretty fun place right now for young adults, and comparatively cheaper than most other locations near the other large London tertiary care centres. In addition, this is one of the few London AFPs (the other ones being at King's) where 2 years are spent at the same hospital. So no faff of another orientation/introduction week and learning all the ins and outs of the hospital. Plus there's a bar in the hospital."

- Dr Xi Ming Zhu - General Practice AFP at St. George's Hospital

"The choice of projects is flexible, you can choose from an extensive list of projects from different specialties - if you know what you want to do a project on this can be arranged."

- Dr Harry Hodgson - Trauma & Orthopaedic Surgery AFP in Yorkshire & Humber

"It can be tough juggling a part-time PGCert course with clinical work, especially with more demanding placements, but it's useful and worth it! Also, being self-motivated and managing your time well during your research block is essential to produce good work!"

- Dr Efioanwan Andah - Primary Care AFP in Yorkshire and Humber

"Organising a swap is much more difficult than I anticipated. I am not very keen on my 3rd rotation of F1 and when applying for the job thought that I would be able to swap it for something that I am more interested in. This has proven to be very difficult!"

- Dr Eyal Ben-David - Renal AFP at St George's Hospital

"My average week in my AFP rotation consists of 3 days of protected research time and 2 days of clinical work at a general practice. Although my AFP is in general practice and my supervisor is an academic GP, my research project is related to ophthalmology and global health. I think if you do want to do your own project, you would have a higher success rate if you plan this early in advance and discuss your idea with your supervisor well in advance of your academic block."

- Dr Saeed Azizi - General Practice AFP at St George's Hospital

5.   What are the most important pieces of advice you would share with an applicant currently applying to the AFP?

"Application: have people who have been through the process to review your white space questions and justify your experiences with the criteria for what makes a good academic doctor.
Academic Interview: Read The Doctor's Guide to Clinical Appraisal! Know all your key terminology inside out, and be confident in how to structure your answers. Know what a Forest plot is, know how ARR differs from RRR, how the different forms of bias can be introduced, how cohort studies differ from case series, etc. The list goes on! It's impossible to learn everything but keep practising your appraisals and present them to friends and colleagues who have some experience in critical appraisal. Most importantly, be confident!
Clinical interview:
(1) DO NOT start with the likely diagnosis – even if it is obvious!
(2) Initially, describe the scenario using the SBAR approach
(3) Work through the patient's case systematically using the ABCDE approach, monitoring all the patient's observations AND assessing the patient's response to any initial management you've offered.
(4) Once you have completed your ABCDE assessment and vocalised this to your interviewers, you are free to give your impression/differential diagnoses. Often the interviewers want a reasonable list of possible differentials.
(5) Then offer your complete management plan – remember to stay within your limits as a Foundation doctor.
(6) The interviewers are looking to ascertain your clinical skills and whether you are situationally aware of your surroundings in clinical practice. That means, seeking help from nursing staff and always escalating to seniors appropriately.
(7) Examiners will often also ask for ongoing management. For example, what is the long-term management of a patient with ACS that you are now looking to discharge?
(8) For all patients, always be aware of who you're going to call and what you can do within your limits of an F1. For example, remember the basics of an upper GI bleed - have a group and save and crossmatch ready, inform the blood bank whilst monitoring and reassessing the patient (delegate tasks to nursing colleagues); remember your other bloods to calculate the patient's Blatchford score (E.g. urea); inform your registrar of the situation and inform the gastro SpR to arrange an urgent endoscopy if indicated.
(9) A general rule of thumb is to offer initial management and stabilise the patient THEN escalate.
(10) For ALL the conditions listed above, learn the basics in terms of risk factors, epidemiology, symptoms, signs, diagnostic criteria (eg. CURB-65, Wells Score, Rockall Score etc), investigations, management, complications, ongoing treatment and prognosis.

(11) When asked about investigations I recommend the BBII approach:

- Bedside (eg full set of observations / ECG / BMs, etc.)
- Bloods (don't forget VBG/ABGs!)
- Imaging (CXR/CT, etc.)
- Intervention (PCI/angiogram, etc.)

(12) REMEMBER: HOW you present a scenario and respond to questions is EQUALLY important as WHAT you say, so ALWAYS speak confidently, clearly, succinctly and maintain good eye contact."

- Dr Azeem Alam - Surgery AFP at St Thomas' Hospital

"If you're going to apply you might as well put in as much effort as you can. It's not worth simply giving it half your effort in the hope you luck out. The application takes place during your final year and you will have many time demands so it's important to prepare well in advance, plan your time and prioritise effectively. Even if you aren't successful, attending the interviews will give you valuable preparation for CT applications"

- Dr Miguel Sequeira Campos - Plastic Surgery AFP at St George's Hospital

"It helps to have an idea of what kind of research or area you are interested in already but this is not essential. It is mostly (with a few exceptions) overestimated how difficult it is to get an AFP post. You don't need a lot of publications or experience but you do need to be able to justify your interest in research: so think about this before your interview "

- Dr Vageesh Jain - Public Health AFP in Leicester

"Be confident and don't hesitate to apply. Focus on being a good doctor and doing research which benefits patients and the rest will follow."

- Dr Shyam Gokani - Primary Care and Population Health AFP at UCL

"Invest time in writing interview preparation and learn it - everyone else you are competing against will be doing this. Practice your interview questions and A->E scenarios with other medical students/doctors. If you are applying to an AFP with white space questions, ensure you have given yourself enough time to redraft them multiple times and get other people to read them and give you feedback. Think of them like mini-personal statements and invest the time you invested into your medical school personal statement."

- Dr Ciaran Kennedy - Medical Education AFP at the University of Sheffield

"Think carefully about your white space questions and contact the careers department at your university as they may do workshops on white space questions or offer interview practice.
It is also very important to think about the clinical rotations on offer. Speak to people who have worked in the hospitals and wards for the five non-academic blocks; these will make up the majority of your foundation years so ensure that you are happy with them."

- Dr Joseph P Thompson - Neurosurgery AFP at Leeds Hospitals Trust

"Use your network to ask for support - with checking white space answers, but most of all with practicing mock interviews.
Make sure that throughout the process you let your character, unique interests and drive come across."

- Dr Rebecca Lissmann - Leadership and Management AFP in South West

"May seem daunting and that your competition is quite stiff, but most people want different things, so chances are if you do well on your interviews, you WILL likely get the AFP that you want."

- Dr Xi Ming Zhu - General Practice AFP at St. George's Hospital

"Don't worry about it too much. It is an exciting opportunity to spend four months doing something you're interested in, but I don't think it's that important if you don't get an AFP job. It won't stop you from embarking on a career in academia if you don't do it as you can still pursue research interests whilst doing the standard FP, and equally you're not committed to a career in academia if you do!"

- Dr Harry Hodgson - Trauma & Orthopaedic Surgery AFP in Yorkshire & Humber

"-Do your research into the academic foundation programmes you want to apply to e.g. what they offer (PGCert course), any extra requirements (I had to email in a separate form with extra information directly to the foundation school alongside my oriel application), how they structure their research placements (4 months vs integrated e.g. 1 day a week over 1 year) - find out all you possibly can!
-Attend AFP preparation and mock interviews courses being offered as they can be useful. One or two should be sufficient as you don't want to overload yourself!
-When it comes to interview, be yourself as that will give you the best platform to be at ease and showcase all the hard work you put into preparing!"

- Dr Efioanwan Andah - Primary Care AFP in Yorkshire and Humber

"Be confident at your interview. Make sure the interviewers know that you are competent and will be a good and safe foundation doctor."

- Dr Eyal Ben-David - Renal AFP at St George's Hospital

"Work hard and work smart, the AFP is really worth it! I know final year can be immensely busy and your time is precious, but you gain plenty from applying and interview itself, as well as the actual AFP itself.
The application processes overlaps with the applications you are likely to complete in the future (ie specialty applications). Completing the application now is likely to make you more conscious of areas of improvement, ie interview skills, research portfolio, CV etc.
Personally, I found my preparation for the AFP clinical stations one of the most helpful experiences in preparing me for F1 as I felt I had to learn my clinical emergencies really well. This consolidated knowledge base gave me more confidence in managing unwell patients as well as knowing when and who to escalate to."

- Dr Saeed Azizi - General Practice AFP at St George's Hospital

6.   What advice would you give to medical students who still have a long time to prepare for the AFP?

"Become a good clinician: Spend time on the wards, learn your medicine, be confident in basic practical skills, attend and observe crash calls, ask questions on ward rounds, go to theatre and really become confident with how a hospital is run. Whilst doing the above, you want to try and become a better researcher. Reach out to potential supervisors. This can be through friends or colleagues that you know, or politely email the corresponding authors of research that interests you. Polite emails offering your assistance in primary or secondary research can get you surprisingly far. Learn how to write effectively, efficiently and succinctly and always stick to deadlines as far as possible. Try to get published and write your own letters to the editor if you are really stuck. Read and write as much as you can. Present posters or speak at local, national and (if you can) international conferences. Speak to other AFP doctors to ensure you are actually interested in academic clinical medicine/surgery. If you can do the above, you are well on your way!"

- Dr Azeem Alam - Surgery AFP at St Thomas' Hospital

"Work hard for your exams; contribute to regular teaching; aim to be well rounded - take part in sports/ hobbies outside of university; aim to publish and present your work; surround yourself with the right people who encourage you to work hard and be better."

- Dr Miguel Sequeira Campos - Plastic Surgery AFP at St George's Hospital

"Get involved in writing - anything, not just peer reviewed publications, but even blogs or less formal things, as it shows interest in a topic and writing is an essential academic skill. If you want to publish, the best way to do it (also the most interesting in my opinion) is to write a commentary or analysis piece on a particular issue. You do usually need some knowledge on this prior but something on medical education or topics of general interest could be an option. Trying to publish from an original research project can be very time consuming, but is definitely useful to explore research interests."

- Dr Vageesh Jain - Public Health AFP in Leicester

"Look at the scoring systems and aim to achieve maximum points in each section. If you start early it is achievable within 2-3 years (apart from higher degrees, etc). Try to do one or two big projects rather than several small projects as this may well be of more value to the scientific community. Remember that the AFP is just the start of the journey and you have a whole medical career to follow. Try to plan a few steps ahead if you can."

- Dr Shyam Gokani - Primary Care and Population Health AFP at UCL

"Start by fretting yourself with your emergency/acute medicine notes and acute management plans. Next move on to preparing the written white space questions/personal statement (if applicable) and consider what presentations, publications and prizes you have attaining and collate evidence of these. You can start thinking about interview questions after you have submitted your written application."

- Dr Ciaran Kennedy - Medical Education AFP at the University of Sheffield

"Try working on your application as early as possible. Projects can take a long time to complete. Submitting abstracts for conferences and submitting manuscripts can be a very lengthy process.
I think there is absolutely no harm in applying, even if you think you may not get a place. You only lose a small amount of time in preparing an application and you may do very well at interview. Even if you don't get a place it's a very valuable application experience going forward."

- Dr Joseph P Thompson - Neurosurgery AFP at Leeds Hospitals Trust

"Find the people who are working on things - publications, audits, quality improvement, presentation or other projects - and ask them whether you can get involved. Simply have a go: The biggest way people lose their power is by giving it away - if you don't apply or ask for something then you definitely won't get it.
Try to gain a little experience in each of the three key areas - research, teaching and leadership."

- Dr Rebecca Lissmann - Leadership and Management AFP in South West

"It's never too early. Many aspects of what determines someone who is a good candidate, especially research, work under a snowball effect."
- Dr Xi Ming Zhu - General Practice AFP at St. George's Hospital

"Ensure you can talk through an A-E assessment and are familiar with the management of common emergencies, and make sure you know how you would succinctly discuss your current research to date and future career plans/goals if asked. Ideally talk to F1 & F2s who have done the interviews and if possible ask if they will do a mock interview for you."
- Dr Harry Hodgson - Trauma & Orthopaedic Surgery AFP in Yorkshire & Humber
"Get involved in research projects you're interested in whilst at medical school - your med school's research/academia society is usually a good place to start. Seek out opportunities to learn from those who have or are doing an AFP to find out what worked for them. Read resources such as this! There's no one size fits all, and everyone's journey will be unique. However, an interest in research/education/leadership should be evident when it comes to applying, even if you don't have a published paper at the time - I didn't!"
- Dr Efioanwan Andah - Primary Care AFP in Yorkshire and Humber

"If you are interested in academia and education then there is no reason not to apply!"
- Dr Eyal Ben-David - Renal AFP at St George's Hospital

"Familiarise yourself with the AFP handbooks and speak to current applicants and those who are currently AFP junior doctors. Form a network early on and I'm sure they'll be delighted to help you along the journey!"
- Dr Saeed Azizi - General Practice AFP at St George's Hospital

7. **What were your top resources when applying for the AFP?**

"1. The Doctor's Guide to Clinical Appraisal
2. Oxford Handbook of Emergency Medicine
3. Medical Interviews: CT, ST and Registrar Interview Skills"
- Dr Azeem Alam - Surgery AFP at St Thomas' Hospital

"Oxford Handbook for Foundation Programme"
- Dr Miguel Sequeira Campos - Plastic Surgery AFP at St George's Hospital

"How to read a paper by Trisha Greenhalgh"
- Dr Vageesh Jain - Public Health AFP in Leicester

"1. Trisha Greenalgh - how to read a paper
2. The Oxford handbook for the foundation programme."
- Dr Shyam Gokani - Primary Care and Population Health AFP at UCL

"I googled 'AFP preparation', bought a couple of AFP books off amazon and read through my emergency medicine medical school notes. What I found most useful was to write my own AFP teaching session powerpoint and then to teach this to myself."
- Dr Ciaran Kennedy - Medical Education AFP at the University of Sheffield

"The careers team at my university (Birmingham) were very good at supporting applicants with workshops and interview practice. These services may be available, but are not always clearly advertised so try to seek them out. There are also a number of very good medical interviews textbooks. These may be for CT or ST interviews, but the interview technique is still transferable."

- Dr Joseph P Thompson - Neurosurgery AFP at Leeds Hospitals Trust

"1. Friends and contacts with academic jobs - advice and interview practice
2. The healthcare careers service - The South West one offers excellent specialist support
3. The Book: 'Medical Interviews, a comprehensive guide'"

- Dr Rebecca Lissmann - Leadership and Management AFP in South West

"1. Oxford Handbook of Clinical Medicine.
2. The Lancet
3. NEJM
4. My two very bright and helpful friends (who got their AFPs too!)"

- Dr Xi Ming Zhu - General Practice AFP at St. George's Hospital

"1. Acute Medicine by Declan O'Kane
2. Oxford Handbook for the Foundation Programme
3. How to Read a Paper by Trisha Greenhalgh

- Dr Harry Hodgson - Trauma & Orthopaedic Surgery AFP in Yorkshire & Humber

"1. Foundation school websites
2. AFP preparation courses e.g. tips on applications and mock interviews
3. Current AFP doctors"

- Dr Efioanwan Andah - Primary Care AFP in Yorkshire and Humber

"1. The New England Journal of Medicine for practicing reading abstracts
2. The Doctors Guide to Critical Appraisal by Gosall and Gosall."

- Dr Eyal Ben-David - Renal AFP at St George's Hospital

"1. Speaking to former / current AFP junior doctors
2. Oxford Handbook of Clinical Medicine
3. Online critical appraisal toolkits / checklists (ie. Cochrane)"

- Dr Saeed Azizi - General Practice AFP at St George's Hospital

Printed in Great Britain
by Amazon

37974150R10066